The Cryptorchid Testis

Editors

Tom O. Abney
Associate Professor
Department of Physiology and Endocrinology
Medical College of Georgia
Augusta, Georgia

Brooks A. Keel
Associate Professor
Department of Obstetrics and Gynecology
University of Kansas School of Medicine — Wichita
The Women's Research Institute
Wichita, Kansas

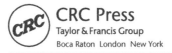

CRC Press
Taylor & Francis Group
Boca Raton London New York

CRC Press is an imprint of the
Taylor & Francis Group, an **informa** business

CRC Press
Taylor & Francis Group
6000 Broken Sound Parkway NW, Suite 300
Boca Raton, FL 33487-2742

© 1989 by Taylor & Francis Group
CRC Press is an imprint of Taylor & Francis Group, an Informa business

First issued in paperback 2019

No claim to original U.S. Government works

ISBN-13: 978-0-367-45099-1 (pbk)
ISBN-13: 978-0-8493-4751-1 (hbk)

Visit the Taylor & Francis Web site at
http://www.taylorandfrancis.com

and the CRC Press Web site at
http://www.crcpress.com

Library of Congress Cataloging-in-Publication Data

The cryptorchid testis.

Includes bibliographies and index.
1. Cryptorchidism—Pathophysiology. I. Abney, Tom O.
II. Keel, Brooks A. [DNLM: 1. Cryptorchidism. 2. Testis—
cytology. WJ 840 C9569]
RJ477.5.C74C78   1989   618.92'68   88-35273
ISBN 0-8493-4751-3

Library of Congress Card Number 88-35273

PREFACE

The idea for this book grew out of discussions between the two editors about the need for a current, comprehensive review of cryptorchidism and the biology of the cryptorchid testis. This book is the result of the combined efforts of a number of internationally known experts in the area of male reproductive biology, each with considerable expertise in the area of cryptorchidism.

In most mammals, the testes descend from an abdominal inguinal location to a scrotal position between the times of birth and sexual maturity. The failure of the testes to descend, either bilaterally or unilaterally, known as cryptorchidism, results in the continued exposure of the male gonad to the higher temperature of the abdomen, as compared to the scrotal temperature. This exposure to increased temperature results in damage to the germinal epithelium and disruption of the normal spermatogenic process. Other cell types are also altered by the abnormal thermal environment and, depending on the duration of the cryptorchid state, irreversible damage can occur. In fact, these thermal induced changes frequently lead to subfertile or infertile males, and often are associated with an increased incidence of testicular cancer. Cryptorchidism occurs in approximately 0.8% of male children and is reported to be increasing in incidence; a sizable number of males are thus affected by this condition. Cryptorchidism is therefore an anomoly with serious long term consequences. Continued investigation of the physiology of testicular descent, the factors involved in maldescent, and the alterations in testicular function that occur as a result of maldescent are thus warranted for a more comprehensive understanding of male reproductive function.

The data and concepts contained in this book and the interpretations presented by the various authors through their individual perspectives offer the reader a wealth of information, and yet pose a number of relevant and interesting questions that must await future research efforts.

THE EDITORS

Tom O. Abney, Ph.D., is Associate Professor in the Department of Physiology and Endocrinology at the Medical College of Georgia in Augusta, Georgia.

Dr. Abney received his B.S. degree in the biological sciences in 1966, and his M.S. and Ph.D. degrees in biochemistry in 1969 and 1972 from the University of Texas in Austin, Texas during 1972 to 1973, and then joined the faculty at the Medical College of Georgia in Augusta in 1973 as Assistant Professor in the Department of Endocrinology.

Dr. Abney's research interest has focused on the endocrine regulation of Leydig cell function, using the rat as a model. He is particularly interested in the role of estrogens in modulating testicular function. In addition, he has conducted studies on Leydig cell function in the cryptorchid animal. He has published over 25 papers in referred journals, and has written chapters in several books related to his studies. His research has received funding from the National Science Foundation, the National Institutes of Health, and Procter and Gamble, Co.

His present research interest concerns the mechanisms which regulate the ontogenic development of Leydig cells.

Brooks A. Keel, Ph.D., is Associate Professor of Obstetrics and Gynecology and Pathology at the University of Kansas School of Medicine — Wichita, and Adjunct Professor of Clinical Sciences at The Wichita State University. Dr. Keel serves as Scientific Director of The Women's Research Institute in Wichita, Kansas.

Dr. Keel received his B.S. degree in biology from Augusta College in 1978 and his Ph.D. in endocrinology from the Medical College of Georgia in 1982. Dr. Keel completed three years of postdoctoral training in reproductive endocrinology at the University of Texas Health Science Center in Houston and the University of South Dakota School of Medicine in Vermillion. He accepted his current position in 1985.

Dr. Keel is a member of the Endocrine Society, the Society for the Study of Reproduction, the American Society of Andrology and the American Fertility Society. He serves on the editorial board for Archives of Andrology and Advances in Contraceptive Delivery Systems. Dr. Keel has published more than forty publications in national and international journals and has served as editor on several books in the area of reproductive endocrinology.

Dr. Keel's research interests include the study of the physiological role and biochemical basis for glycoprotein heterogeneity, and the mechanisms controlling pituitary-testicular function. His grant support is from the Wesley Medical Research Institutes, the Women's Research Institute, and the National Institutes of Health.

CONTRIBUTORS

Tom O. Abney
Associate Professor
Department of Physiology and
  Endocrinology
Medical College of Georgia
Augusta, Georgia

Anders R. J. Bergh
Associate Professor
Department of Pathology
University of Umea
Umea, Sweden

David M. de Kretser
Professor
Department of Anatomy
Monash University
Clayton, Victoria, Australia

Momokazu Gotoh
Research Associate
Department of Urology
Nagoya University School of Medicine
Nagoya, Japan

H. Edward Grotjan, Jr.
Associate Professor
Department of Animal Science
University of Nebraska
Lincoln, Nebraska

Friedrich Jockenhovel
Research Fellow
Division of Endocrinology
Department of Medicine
Harbor-UCLA Medical Center
Torrance, California

Brooks A. Keel
Associate Professor
Department of Obstetrics and Gynecology
University of Kansas School of Medicine
  — Wichita
The Women's Research Institute
Wichita, Kansas

Jeffrey B. Kerr
Department of Anatomy
Monash University
Clayton, Victoria, Australia

Larry I. Lipshultz
Professor
Scott Department of Urology
Baylor College of Medicine
Houston, Texas

Hideo Mitsuya
Professor
Department of Urology
Nagoya University School of Medicine
Nagoya, Japan

Koji Miyake
Professor and Chairman
Department of Urology
Nagoya University School of Medicine
Nagoya, Japan

Gail P. Risbridger
Senior Research Officer
Department of Anatomy
Monash University
Clayton, Victoria, Australia

David R. Roth
Assistant Professor
Scott Department of Urology
Baylor College of Medicine
Houston, Texas

Bruce D. Schanbacher
Reproduction Research Unit
United States Department of Agriculture
Clay Center, Nebraska

Richard M. Sharpe
MRC Reproductive Biology Unit
Centre for Reproductive Biology
Edinburgh, Scotland

Ronald S. Swerdloff
Professor and Chief
Division of Endocrinology
Department of Medicine
UCLA School of Medicine
Los Angeles, California

TABLE OF CONTENTS

Chapter 1

OVERVIEW OF CRYPTORCHIDISM WITH EMPHASIS ON THE HUMAN

David R. Roth and Larry I. Lipshultz

TABLE OF CONTENTS

I. INTRODUCTION

Few problems in clinical urology are likely to span as many years and require as much attention of other specialists as cryptorchid testes. The problem has been recognized for thousands of years; yet we are just now beginning to understand its causes, its intrinsic effect on the testes, and its implications with regard to both fertility and malignant degeneration. The available data are further confused by the occasional inclusion, often unintentional, of the retractile rather than truly cryptorchid testis. Additionally, the effects of treatment, whether with surgery or hormonal manipulation, are difficult to assess, especially since the cryptorchid testis may represent a potentially dysgenetic organ.

The authors will, in this chapter, examine some of the basic concepts pertaining to potential subfertility and cryptorchidism. A review of the basic embryology, anatomy, and mechanisms of testicular descent is followed by a discussion of the classification and incidence of maldescent. Finally, the effects of maldescent are described and the relationship of gonadal dysfunction and resultant subfertility are explored.

II. EMBRYOLOGY

A. Urogenital Ridge

The urogenital ridge first appears in the 4th week of gestation as paired ridges on the posterior abdomen just lateral to the dorsal midline. It is composed of two adjacent structures: the medial genital ridge and the lateral mesonephric ridge. These develop in a caudal direction and ultimately give rise to lateral mesonephric kidneys and the medially located undifferentiated gonads (Figure 1).

B. The Undifferentiated Gonad

The primordial gonad is a mass of mesoderm which will subsequently differentiate into the somatic elements of the gonad. The germinal components (primordial germ cells or gonocytes) arising in the 4th week of embryonic life are derived from the entoderm of the posterior aspect of the yolk sac and thus have an extragonadal origin. These gonocytes migrate laterally by ameboid action along the side walls of the forming gut, then move through its mesentery to ultimately rest upon the developing genital ridges (Figure 2). The gonocytes proliferate during this migration and complete their journey by the 6th week of gestation.

C. Gonadal Differentiation

Differentiation of the primordial gonads into either ovaries or testes begins after arrival of the gonocytes at the genital ridge. Differentiation into a testis is regulated by the expression of the H-Y antigen as determined by the Y chromosome. This surface antigen promotes the organization of the gonadal blastema into a recognizable testis.

The interstitium of the testes is then carved into a series of arched, branched, and anastomotic sex cords by the ingrowth at the hilus of mesenchyme and blood vessels. The primordial germ cells are sequestered within these developing sex cords, and the mesenchymal elements accompanying the gonocytes develop into Sertoli cells. The sex cells are further defined by a basal lamina and surrounding mesenchenyma. Those mesenchymal elements, not part of the sex cords, differentiate into the interstitium and Leydig cells.

The rete testes are formed from smaller cords at the edge of the sex cords and are directed towards the testicular hilus. Gonocytes outside the sex cords, within the rete cords or interstitium, perish. The mesenchyme at the periphery of the gonad coalesces to form the tunica albuginea, and by the 8th week of gestation a recognizable testis has developed.

The mesenephros, just lateral to the genital ridge, begins to regress at about this same

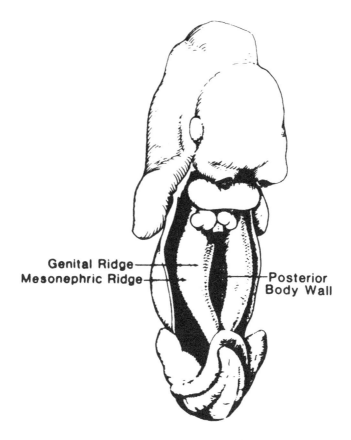

FIGURE 1. View of the posterior abdominal wall in a young embryo. The genital and mesonephric ridges lie on either side of the dorsal midline, and together form the urogenital ridge. (From Arey, L. B., *Developmental Anatomy*, 7th ed., W. B. Saunders, Philadelphia, 1974. With permission.)

time. Most mesonephric tubules degenerate, leaving 12 to 15 that abut upon the testicular hilus. These few tubules grow toward the testis, establish continuity with the rete cords and eventually become the ductuli efferentes. These tubules maintain their continuity with the mesonephric or Wolffian Duct which develops into the vas deferens and epididymis (Figure 3).

D. Leydig Cells

Fetal Leydig cells begin to differentiate in the 8th week of development and soon begin to secrete steroids. The peak production of testosterone occurs in the 12th week. This production stimulates differentiation of the epididymis, vas deferens, accessory glands, and external genitalia. During the 5th month of gestation, these Leydig cells disappear (either degenerate or dedifferentiate) and testosterone levels fall. Leydig cells then reemerge at the time of puberty.

E. Sertoli Cell Development

The Sertoli cells proliferate after spermatogenesis has begun and fuse with tight junctional complexes to form an impermeable membrane to blood (Figure 4). This blood/testis barrier establishes a basal and adluminal compartment within the seminferous tubule. Spermatogenesis begins within the basal compartment. Once DNA synthesis is complete, the tight Sertoli cell junctions separate transiently to allow the leptotene spermatocytes to enter the

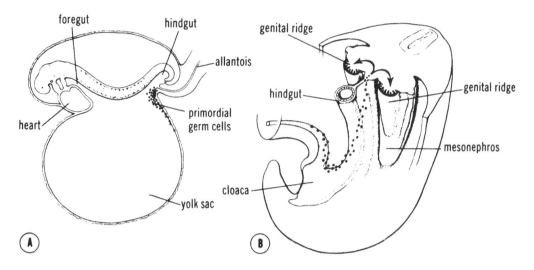

FIGURE 2.   (A) Schematic drawing of a 3-week-old embryo showing the primordial germ cells in the wall of the yolk sac, close to the attachment of the allantois (after Witchi). (B) Drawing showing the migration path of the primordial germ cells along the wall of the hindgut and the dorsal mesentery into the genital ridge. Note the position of the genital ridge and mesonephros. (From Langman, J., *Medical Embryology*, Williams & Wilkins, Baltimore, 1969, 165. With permission.)

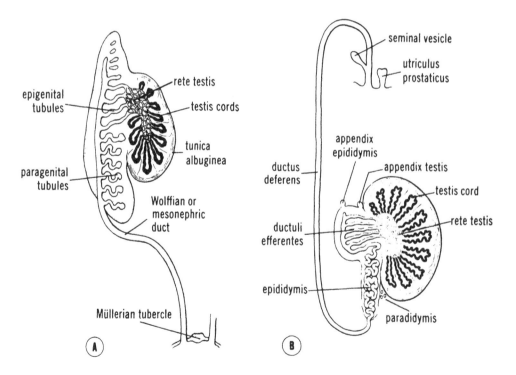

FIGURE 3.   (A) Diagram of the genital ducts in the male in the 4th month of development. The Mullerian duct has degenerated except for the appendix testis and the utriculus prostaticus. (B) The genital duct after descent of the testis. Note the horseshoe-shaped testis cords, the rete testis, and the ductuli efferentes entering the ductus deferens. The paradidymis is formed by the remnants of the paragenital mesonephric tubules. (From Langman, J., *Medical Embryology*, Williams & Wilkins, Baltimore, 1969, 169. With permission.)

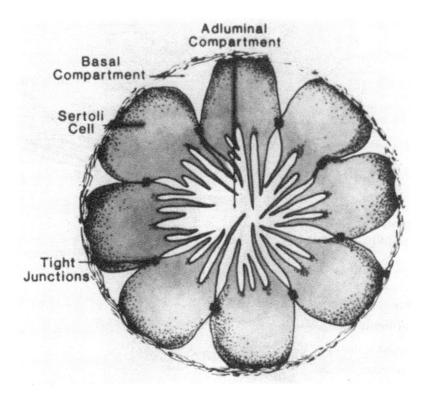

FIGURE 4. Structure of the tubular wall in the absence of germ cells. The blood-testis barrier forms at the level of the tight junctions. (From Huckins, C., *Infertility in the Male*, Lipshultz, L. I. and Howards, S. S., Eds., Churchill Livingstone, New York, 1983, 12. With permission.)

luminal compartment and further differentiate into spermatocytes. This unique luminal environment is essential for further development of the spermatocytes. The blood/testis barrier develops rather late and has not been observed in humans under 11 years of age; it appears to be hormonally regulated by FSH.

III. ANATOMY

A. Description of Testes

The adult testes are a pair of oval organs measuring 4 to 5 cm in length and 2.25 cm in width and weighing 10.5 to 14 g. The testes lie upright in the scrotum with the long axis tilted slightly forward and lateral. The posterior aspect of the testis is attached to the epididymis which leads to the vas deferens (Figure 5).

B. Tunica Vaginalis

The processus vaginalis is an outpouching of the fetal peritoneum from which the tunica vaginalis is derived. The processus vaginalis precedes the testes during its descent into the scrotum. The proximal portion of the processus vaginalis obliterates, whereas the portion distal to the external ring, the tunica vaginalis, remains patent, enveloping the testes and epididymis. The inner visceral layer covers the testis, epididymis, and distal spermatic cord. The outer or parietal layer is well attached to the other coverings of the testis and lines the scrotal chamber. The sac between these two layers normally contains a small amount of fluid and pathologically forms a hydrocele. If the processus vaginalis does not obliterate, a patent processus vaginalis or congenital hernia results.

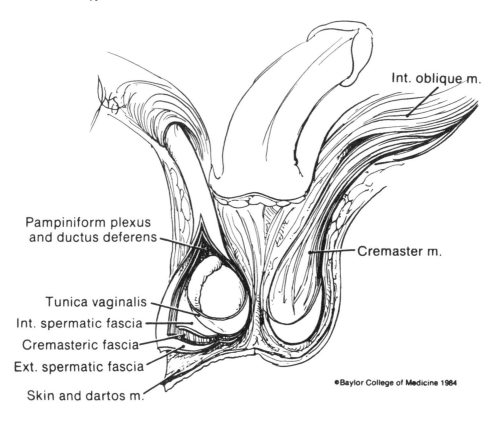

FIGURE 5.   Dissection of scrotal contents, illustrating the coverings of the testis. (From Meacham, R. B., Huckins, C., and Lipshultz, L. I., in *Principles and Management of Testicular Cancer,* Thieme-Stratton, New York, 1986, 14. With permission.)

C. Epididymis

The epididymis is a curved structure approximately 5 cm in length on the posterior lateral aspect of the testes. It has been divided into three portions. The globus major, or head, of the epididymis is firmly attached to the superior aspect of the testis by the efferent ductules. The corpus, or body, lies upon the posterior portion of the testis but is separated from it. The globus minor, or tail, of the epididymis is loosely attached to the testis and leads to the vas deferens. The ductuli efferent perforate' the tunica albuginea of the testes and then proceed to the globus major where they enter the epididymis (Figure 6).

D. Testes

The parenchyme of the testes is covered by a dense inelastic covering consisting of interlacing bundles of fibrous tissue known as the tunica albuginea. The inner aspect of this structure gives off several thin septae which converge to form the mediastinum of the testes. This complex supports the blood vessels and ducts of the gonad. The septae form several wedges which are wide at the periphery and narrow as they converge upon the mediastinum. It is estimated that there are 250 to 400 lobules in each testis. The arteries, veins, and lymphatics enter the posterior aspect of the testes, then transverse the mediastinum and spread out on the inner surface of the mediastinum to form the tunica vasculosa.

Within each tubule lie the parenchyma of the testis consisting of the seminiferous tubules. There are an estimated 840 tubules per testis, each one with an average length of 70 to 80 cm and diameter of 0.12 to 0.30 mm. These tubules converge upon the mediastinum where they become less convoluted and join other tubules to form from 20 to 30 larger tubuli recti

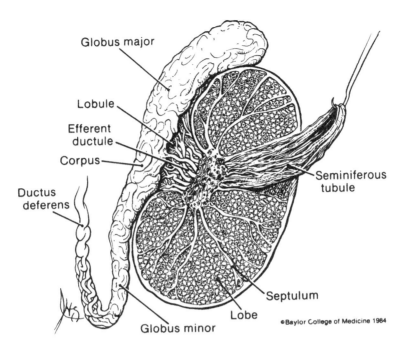

Globus major

Lobule

Efferent
ductule

Corpus

Ductus
deferens

Seminiferous
tubule

Septulum

Lobe

Globus minor

©Baylor College of Medicine 1984

FIGURE 6. Cross-sectional representative of the testis and epididymis. (From Meacham, R. B., Huckins, C., and Lipshultz, L. I., in *Principles and Management of Testicular Cancer*, Thieme-Stratton, New York, 1986, 15. With permission.)

which are 0.5 mm in diameter. Within the mediastinum they coalesce to form epithelial-lined channels known as the rete testis. The rete testis terminate with 12 to 20 ductuli efferentes which perforate the tunica albuginea and proceed to the epididymis.

E. Arterial Supply

The arterial supply to the testes consists of three vessels. The largest vessel is the internal spermatic artery which arises directly from the aorta and parallels the ureter into the pelvis, passing through the internal ring with the spermatic cord to end upon the posterior aspect of the testes.

The deferential artery originates from the interior vesicle artery and travels closely approximated with the vas deferens until it reaches the globus minor where it branches into a capillary network. The third artery, the external spermatic or cremasteric artery, originates from the inferior epigastric artery, passes through the inguinal canal within the sheath of the cord, and continues to the parietal surface of the tunica vaginalis where it anastamoses with capillaries from the other vessels (Figure 7).

IV. MALDESCENT

A. Mechanism of Testicular Descent

Since Hunter's treatise in 1841,[1] many theories have been proposed to explain testicular descent. These have included gubernacular tension pulling the testes into the scrotum, Cleland's theory of differential growth,[2] and an increase in intraabdominal pressure.[1,3,4] As early as 1932, an endocrine-mediated event was suggested. Engle showed that early descent could be induced in monkeys treated with either a water-soluble anterior pituitary extract of urine from pregnant monkeys.[5] Further studies with both animals and humans have pointed towards testosterone as the hormonal mediator.[6] Further delineation was added by Rajfer in 1977 when he suggested that dihydrotestosterone rather than testosterone may be the active

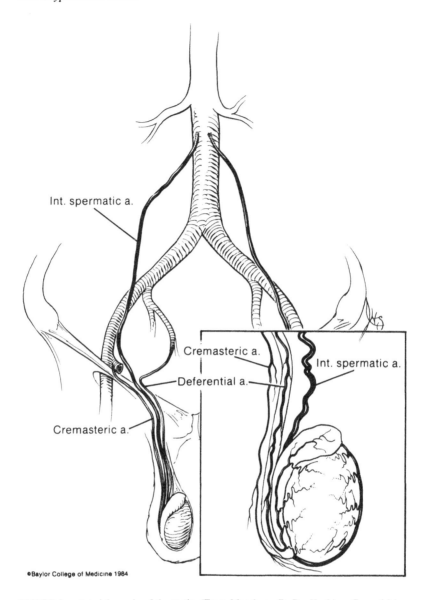

FIGURE 7.   Arterial supply of the testis. (From Meacham, R. B., Huckins, C., and Lip-shultz, L. I., in *Principles and Management of Testicular Cancer,* Thieme-Stratton, New York, 1986, 17. With permission.)

metabolite.[7] Moreover, the dihydrotestosterone must be present locally in high concentration within the testes for the hormone to influence descent. The exact mechanism of its action remains to be fully delineated.

Current data from rodent experiments suggest that the process of testicular descent may not be solely dependent upon any one system but rather is related to a combination of intraabdominal pressure,[8] the integrity of the gubernaculum,[9] and hormonal influences.[7] Deficiency of any one element may lead to an aberration of testicular descent.

B. Classification of Maldescent

Before one can adequately discuss the effect of maldescent one must define the various degrees of cryptorchidism. A classic categorization was proposed by Scorer and Farrington in 1971 and is the basis for the diagram in Figure 8.[10]

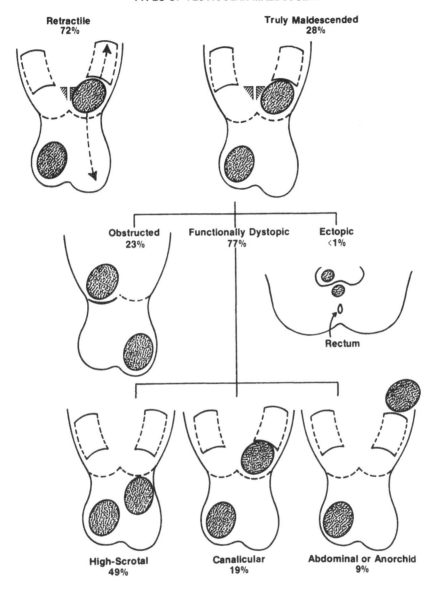

FIGURE 8.   Types of testicular maldescent. (From Lipshultz, L. I., *Fertil. Steril.*, 27, 610, 1976. With permission.)

In the schema the retractile testis is included only for completeness. In fact, a retractile testis, one which can be easily brought into the scrotum and will stay there for a short while, is thought to belong in a separate category and require no further treatment. This form of dystopia is the most common encountered, accounting for between 50 and 80% of referrals for maldescent problems.[10-13] The testis retracts into the superficial inguinal pouch by the action of a hyperactive cremasteric muscle. Furthermore, this group of subjects must be identified in any series which comments on either spontaneous testicular descent or fertility after cryptorchidism since these gonads have both normal descent and fertility.

The other categories represent truly undescended testes and are based upon placement of the gonad. Scorer divides these patients into those with obstructed testes (23%), those with functionally dystopic testes (77%), and those with ectopic testes (1%). The obstructed testes are those which become trapped by adjacent tissue along the normal pathway. There is no apparent failure of the mechanism of descent. The ectopic group are those organs which have gotten off their usual pathway and reside in an unusual extrascrotal/extragonadal location, such as the thigh, suprapubic regions, or perineum.

The largest dystopic group consists of those gonads which exhibit failure of descent yet are unobstructed and found along the normal course of downward migration. Scorer divides these functionally dystopic testes into three categories — intraabdominal (9%), canicular (19%), or high scrotal (49%).[10] A fourth category has been defined by Hadziselmovic.[13] He described the gliding testis, i.e., one which can be manipulated into the scrotum but which returns immediately after release to the superficial inguinal pouch. The significance of a gliding testes, he suggests, is that these represent the best candidates for hormonal treatment of maldescent.[13]

C. Incidence of Undescended Testes

The reported incidence of maldescent reflects many inconsistencies and contradictions. Clearly there is an increased incidence of maldescent in premature infants, and this is dependent upon the degree of prematurity. Scorer (1971) reported an incidence of undescent in full-term boys to be 3.4%,[10] whereas Hadziselmovic reported an incidence of 5.83%.[13] In his series, Scorer described a spontaneous descent as one occurring any time from the first weeks to the third or fourth month of life. This spontaneous descent is thought to be related to a transient rise in testosterone in the first several months of life. The incidence of maldescent at 1 year of age was between 0.7[14] and 1.8%,[13] a level approximately equal to that in untreated adults.

D. Infertility and Maldescent

As early as the 18th century, Hunter recognized the association between cryptorchidism and infertility and stated his belief that when one or both testes remain through life in the belly, they are "exceedingly imperfect and probably incapable of performing their normal function."[1]

Elevated extrascrotal temperature has been shown to be detrimental to spermatogenesis in the affected testis (see Chapter 9); however, a more general effect is suggested by the fact that individuals with *unilateral* cryptorchidism have a significant incidence of infertility, i.e., a bilateral effect. Unfortunately, the precise frequency of infertility associated with cryptorchidism is difficult to quantify. Few series mention whether retractile gonads were excluded or document the location of the testes prior to treatment. Furthermore, because the data are often drawn from a population who have infertility problems, data from infertility clinics obviously are biased, and thus exert a negative influence. The incidence of cryptorchidism in the general population is about 1%; much higher rates (8.3%) have been reported in patients being seen in an infertility clinic.[15] A full 20% of the azoospermic population in the study reported by David had a history of cryptorchidism.[15] Screening for various syndromes such as prune belly syndrome variants, intersex, and Klinefelter's syndrome are seldom mentioned; yet inclusion of men with these disorders would have a significant impact because these patients are universally infertile.

It is clear that progressive testicular injury occurs as the testis remains extrascrotal. Yet most series either fail to stratify patients in terms of age at the time of treatment or will group the patients in categories encompassing many years. Such large groupings may mask subtle differences and, more importantly, ignore the current trend of early surgical or hormonal treatment, i.e., less than 18 months. Data reflecting the efficacy of early therapy are not yet available because many children who had early intervention have not yet reached adulthood. Very early treatment possibly may exert a beneficial effect upon fertility.[16]

A second potentially important influence is the effect of human chorionic gonadotropin (hCG) treatment on subsequent fertility. It has been suggested that those individuals who respond positively to a series of hCG injections have better fertility than those who have failed hormonal therapy and have subsequently undergone an orchiopexy. This finding may be attributable to a more severe form of cryptorchidism and testicular dysfunction in the latter group. Hence, those individuals who have received hCG must be identified and separated accordingly.[17]

Some investigators have attempted to correlate the preintervention gonadal location with a histologic technique termed the "tubule fertility index" (TFI). The TFI (percent of testicular tubules containing spermatogonia) of undescended testes increases as the testicular position approximates the scrotum.[10] Therefore, it is imperative to categorize patients by testicular position and report results accordingly.

The retractile testes must be addressed separately. It has been shown that retractile testes develop normally and produce normal fertility rates.[18] Therefore, attempts must be made and documented to exclude patients with retractile testes from the cryptorchid series. Despite these efforts, exclusion of patients with retractile testes may be difficult because of the subtlety of physical findings and variation among different examiners.

Epididymal abnormalities have been reported to occur in approximately one third of children with undescended testes.[19,20] In the studies by Heath and Marshall, these abnormalities ranged from complete absence of the epididymis and vas to a normal attachment of the head and tail with very loose attachment of the body (See Figure 9). The incidence of epididymal abnormalities was dependent upon whether the testis was ectopic (21%), undescended with a complete hernia sac (75%), or undescended without a complete hernia sac (16%).[19] Yet most operative reports fail to note epididymal anatomy which could affect subsequent fertility. Furthermore, any series incorporating hormonal treatment will miss those individuals who may be subfertile because of anatomic anomalies rather than testicular dysfunction.

Various series addressing the problem of infertility after orchiopexy neglect the problems of surgical injury and subsequent atrophy, inadequate post-operative position, or possible vasal injury, estimated to be as high as 2%.[21] Hadziselimovic reported that normal testes which have ascended after a herniorrhaphy show progressive injury; after 10 years in an unfavorable extrascrotal position, these testes will exhibit atrophic intra-tubular changes.[22] Sertoli cells and spermatogonia show pyknotic nuclei and cytoplasmsic vacuoles. Therefore, in the patient treated surgically for cryptorchidism, the final position of the testis should be assessed and operative results reviewed to identify possible sugical injury.

Fertility data generally are collated on the basis of either sperm analysis or paternity. Each method has inherent difficulties. Sperm analysis requires attention to such criteria as number and variability in specimens obtained and period of abstinence required prior to collection; both variables may introduce error into the final data tabulation. Data relating to sperm function often are not available, yet may have a significant impact on fertility. Paternity as a measure of fertility may not truly reflect the extent of testicular damage and must be evaluated with this in mind.

Evidence for a bilateral defect in the individual with unilateral testicular maldescent has its basis in the studies previously mentioned and in mammalian studies as well. Experimental studies in rats with unilateral acquired cryptorchidism have shown an effect in the contralateral gonad. It is tempting to postulate an immunologic basis for this contralateral injury, yet it has been difficult to prove definitely. Exciting work has been performed by Kogan and associates in which rats with unilateral acquired cryptorchidism have been shown to have decreased fertility when compared to controls as measured by litter size.[23] Of course, one must always be cautioned in extrapolating rodent data directly to the human.

Kogan gathered data from 11 recent series of patients with unilateral cryptorchidism and 9 series of patients with bilateral cryptorchidism. He reported sperm density greater than 20

EPIDIDYMAL ABNORMALITY

A. A Agenesis of epididymis-vas deferens

B. Atresia, loss of continuity between:
1. Head of epididymis and testis

2. Mid-epididymis

3. Tail of epididymis

C. Loop or Elongated Epididymis

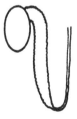

FIGURE 9. Classification of epididymal abnormalities. (Modified from Marshall, F. F. and Shermeta, D. W., Epididymal abnormalities associated with undescended testis, *J. Urol.*, 121, 342, 1979. With permission.)

million/cc in only 51.5% (range 25 to 81%) of 561 men with a history of unilateral cryptorchidism. Therefore, it is apparent that even a unilateral abnormality is reflected in decreased sperm count in a significant number of patients.[24] Of 281 men with a history of bilateral undescended testes, only 28% (range 8 to 48%) had a normal sperm count.[24] However, these findings are not universal. Gilhooly stated that fertility in patients after an orchiopexy for unilateral cryptorchidism was not different from that of the general population,[25] and Fallon reported similar results.[26]

Two recent studies using sperm density[27,28] have suggested that there is no ipsilateral sperm production after an orchiopexy. They both investigated adults who had undergone unilateral orchiopexy and later returned for vasectomy. Unilateral vasectomy was done on the contralateral side and semen analysis performed. Evaluation uniformly showed decreased sperm counts, implying significant testicular dysfunction. Both of these studies included individuals who, for the most part, had had orchiopexies after age 6.

Other authors have suggested that orchiopexy before age 2 will offer the best opportunity for preservation of testicular function.[29] Gaudio documented changes in testicular histology as early as 2 years of age and observed ultrastructural abnormalities in the Sertoli cell in patients of this age as well.[30] Hadziselimovic found that 22% of 2-year-olds with unilateral cryptorchidism had already lost all germ cells in the ipsilateral testis.[22] Those testes with germ cells present showed inhibition of development. Significantly, the contralateral gonad showed a definite decrease in the germ cell population when compared to uninvolved control gonads.

It appears, therefore, that definite morphological changes occur in the cryptorchid testis within the first 2 years of life. If we hope to alter the significant degree of hypofertility present in those individuals with unilateral as well as bilateral cryptorchidism, we must intervene either hormonally or surgically prior to the advent of identifiable damage.

REFERENCES

1. **Hunter, J. A.,** A description of the situation of the testis in the fetus with its descent into the scrotum, in *Observations on Certain Parts of the Animal Oeconomy,* John J. Haswell, New Orleans, 1841.
2. **Alojzy, M.,** Significance of biopsy research in cryptorchidism in children, *Arch. Dis. Child.,* 38, 170, 1963.
3. **Gier, H. T. and Marion, G.,** Development of the mammalian testes by the anterior pituitary-like principle, *N.Y. State J. Med.,* 36, 15, 1936.
4. **Rajfer, J. and Walsh, P. C.,** Testicular descent normal and abnormal, *Urol. Clin. N. Am.,* 5, 223, 1978.
5. **Engle, E. T.,** Experimentally induced descent of the testis in the *Macacus* monkey by hormones from the anterior pituitary and pregnancy urine, *Endocrinology,* 16, 513, 1932.
6. **Martins, T.,** Mechanism of the descent of the testicle under the actions of sex hormones, in *Essays in Biology,* Simpson, M. E., Ed., University of California Press, Berkeley, 1943.
7. **Rajfer, J. and Walsh, P. C.,** Hormonal regulation of testicular descent: experimental and clinical observations, *J. Urol.,* 118, 985, 1977.
8. **Kaplan, L. M., Koyle, M. A., Kaplan, G. W., Farrer, J. H., and Rajfer, J.,** Association between abdominal wall defects and cryptorchidism, *J. Urol.,* 136, 645, 1986.
9. **Frey, H. L. and Rajfer, J.,** Role of the gubernaculum and intraabdominal pressure in the process of testicular descent, *J. Urol.,* 131, 574, 1984.
10. **Scorer, C. G. and Farrington, G. H.,** *Congenital Deformities of the Testis and Epididymis,* Butterworth's, London, 1971, chap. 3.
11. **Lipshultz, L. I., Caminos-Torres, R., Greenspan, C. S., and Snyder, P. J.,** Testicular function after orchiopexy for unilaterally undescended testis, *N. Engl. J. Med.,* 295, 15, 1976.
12. **Scorer, C. G. and Farrington, G. H.,** Congenital anomalies of the testes, in *Campbell's Urology,* 4th ed., Harrison, J. H., Gittes, R. F., Perlmutter, A. D., et al., Eds., W. B. Saunders, Philadelphia, 1979, chap. 44.
13. **Hadziselimovic, F.,** Examination and clinical findings in cryptorchid boys, in *Cryptorchidism, Management and Implications,* Hadziselimovic, F., Ed., Springer-Verlag, Berlin, 1983, chap. 8.
14. **Scorer, C. G. and Farrington, G. H.,** Failure of testicular descent, in *Congenital Deformities of the Testis and Epididymis,* Butterworth's, London, 1971, chap. 2.
15. **David, G., Bisson, J. P., Martin-Boyce, A., and Feneux, D.,** Sperm characteristics and fertility in previously cryptorchid adults, in *Cryptorchidism, Diagnosis and Treatment,* Vol. 6, Job, Jean-Claude, Ed., S. Karger, New York, 1979, 187.
16. **Giarola, A. and Agostini, G.,** Undescended testis and male infertility, *Proc. Int. Symp. on Cryptorchidism,* Bierich, J. R. and Giarola, A., Eds., Academic Press, New York, 1978, 533.

17. **Knorr, D.,** Fertility after HCG-treatment of maldescended testes, in *Cryptorchidism, Diagnosis and Treatment,* Vol. 6, Job, Jean-Claude, Ed., S. Karger, New York, 1979, 215.

18. **Puri, P. and Nixon, H H.,** Bilateral retractile testes — subsequent effects on fertility, *J. Pediatr. Surg.,* 12, 563, 1977.

19. **Heath, A. L., Man, D. W. K., and Eckstein, H. B.,** Epididymal abnormalities associated with maldescent of the testis, *J. Pediatr., Surg.,* 19(1), 47, 1984.

20. **Marshall, F. F. and Shermeta, D. W.,** Epididymal abnormalities associated with undescended testis, *J. Urol.,* 121, 341, 1979.

21. **Mengel, W. and Hecker, W. C.,** Cryptorchidism — surgical treatment and its date, in *Cryptorchidism, Diagnosis and Treatment,* Vol. 6, Job, Jean-Claude, Ed., S. Karger, New York, 1979, 160.

22. **Hadziselimovic, F.,** Histology and ultrastructure of normal and cryptorchid testes, in *Cryptorchidism, Management and Implications,* Hadziselimovic, F., Ed., Springer-Verlag, Berlin, 1983, chap. 4.

23. **Juenemann, K-P., Kogan, B. A., and Abozeid, M. H.,** Fertility in cryptorchidism: an experimental model, *J. Urol.,* 136, 214, 1986.

24. **Kogan, S. J.,** Fertility in cryptorchidism, in *Cryptorchidism, Management and Implications,* Hadziselimovic, F., Ed., Springer-Verlag, Berlin, 1983, chap. 6.

25. **Gilhooly, P. E., Meyers, F., and Lattimer, J. K.,** Fertility prospects for children with cryptorchidism, *Am. J. Dis. Childr.,* 138, 940, 1984.

26. **Fallon, B. and Kennedy, T. J.,** Long-term follow-up of fertility in cryptorchid patients, *Urology,* 25(5), 502, 1985.

27. **Alpert, P. F. and Klein, R. S.,** Spermatogenesis in the unilateral cryptorchid testis after orchiopexy, *J. Urol.,* 129, 301, 1983.

28. **Eldrup, J. and Steven, K.,** Influence of orchiopexy for cryptorchidism on subsequent fertility, *Br. J. Surg.,* 67, 269, 1980.

29. **Molnar, D., Leb, J., Hidvegi, J., and Papp, G.,** Follow-up examination of patients with undescended testicles, *Acta Paediatr. Acad. Sci. Hung.,* 22, 177, 1981.

30. **Gaudio, E., Paggiarino, D., and Carpino, F.,** Structural and ultrastructural modifications of cryptorchid human testes, *J. Urol.,* 131, 292, 1984.

Chapter 2

EXPERIMENTAL MODELS OF CRYPTORCHIDISM

Anders R. J. Bergh

TABLE OF CONTENTS

I. INTRODUCTION

Cryptorchidism is the single most common malformation in human males as well as in several other mammalian species.[1-3] The incidence in man is 1.4 to 2.7%, and it is probably increasing.[4] Cryptorchidism results in impaired fertility and an increased risk of testicular cancer, but the mechanisms responsible are only partially understood. Spermatogenesis cannot take place at abdominal temperatures, but the cellular mechanisms involved and the evolutionary advantage of this unique temperature sensitivity are unknown.[5-7] To what extent the morphological and functional changes in a cryptorchid testis are reversible has not been fully established.

In order to gain knowledge on the pathophysiology of cryptorchidism, a myriad of investigators, starting with Griffiths 94 years ago,[8] have been using experimentally cryptorchid testes in order to imitate the congenital condition. Experimental cryptorchidism can be induced in several ways using different species and the number of studies using experimental cryptorchidism is very large and all aspects of this topic cannot be reviewed here. In this chapter, I have chosen to present and compare different experimental models of cryptorchidism, particularly those used in rats. However, before going into that and before discussing advantages and disadvantages of different models, it must be realized that different investigators use experimentally cryptorchid animals for different reasons. The principal aim is sometimes not to mimic the congenital condition and thereby elucidate the pathophysiology of that condition in particular. Instead, for example, experimental cryptorchidism may be used as a way to induce a particular type of testicular damage and study the effect on the regulation of gonadotrophin secretion. All cell types in the testis are not sensitive to abdominal temperatures per se, but, after some time of experimental cryptorchidism, the functions of almost all cell types in the testis are affected. Experimental cryptorchidism may thus be used as a model to study cell-cell interactions in the testis. Using different types of experimentally cryptorchid testes, more general and extremely valuable information concerning testicular physiology and pathophysiology have been obtained. However, as will be discussed below, the data obtained in one experimental model cannot always be directly applied to another and the results may sometimes be of limited value when trying to understand the pathophysiology of congenital cryptorchidism. The aim of this review is to emphasize that there are several types of "experimentally cryptorchid testes" with different morphologies and functions. Some of these mimic the congenital condition more than others, but they all may provide important information depending on the aim.

II. SURGICALLY INDUCED EXPERIMENTAL CRYPTORCHIDISM

A. In Adult Rats

The most common method for inducing cryptorchidism is to reposition descended testes in adult animals by cutting the gubernaculum testis and moving the testis back into the abdominal cavity. Redescent is prevented either by suturing the testis to the abdominal wall or by closing the inguinal canal. It is generally assumed that these methods give identical results, but no systematic comparative study is available. On the contrary, indirect evidence suggests that the effect on the testis may be slightly different. Testis weight is probably the single most informative parameter of testis function. Upon reviewing a number of studies using these two methods in adult rats, it appears that there is often, but not always, a larger decrease in testis weight when the testis is sutured to the abdominal wall compared to when the inguinal canal is closed (Table 1). After unilateral cryptorchidism for 4 weeks, the average weight of the abdominal testis is reduced to 28 and 35% of that in the scrotal testis, respectively. A similar difference between models may also be present in bilateral cryptorchidism, the average testis weight is reduced to 32 and 38%, respectively.[9-16] This comparison

Table 1
EFFECT OF EXPERIMENTAL CRYPTORCHIDISM ON
UNILATERAL ABDOMINAL TESTES WEIGHTS

.nguinal canal closed	Ref.	Testis sutured to the abdominal wall	Ref.
		0.28 g — 17%	140
0.701 g — 35%	138		
0.467 g — 28%	96	0.44 g — 26%	13
0.66 g — 41%	16		
0.63 g — 38%	139	0.57 g — 24%	98
0.53 g — 33%	93	0.691 g — 43%	141

Note: Data were obtained from adult rats, rendered cryptorchid for 4 weeks. Data are expressed as the absolute weights (grams) and as percent of the scrotal testes.

does obviously not prove that these two methods give different results, it only indicates that some precaution is needed when data obtained in one model is used in another. There is also considerable variation within the groups (Table 1). In absolute terms, the size of the abdominal testis in one study may be twice as large as in another using the same experimental model and duration (Table 1). It would not be surprising if testis function is different in these studies. The reason for these differences within and between groups is unknown, but the variability suggests that the models are not sufficiently characterized. One explanation for differences may be that the temperature in the abdominal cavity is not uniform, as discussed already by Moore and Quick,[17,18] but other factors may also be of importance. When the inguinal canal is closed, some investigators have reported problems with partial or complete redescent when the sutures are resorbed.[15] This may explain reports of spontaneous recovery of spermatogenesis in some abdominal testes.[19] Moreover, Gunn et al.[20] claimed that there are differences in morphology in the caudal and cranial poles of the testis in rats made cryptorchid by suturing the inguinal canal. In this experimental model, the testis is lying freely movable in the lower part of the abdominal cavity. Its vascular pedicle may, at least theoretically, be torsioned-retorsioned, but whether this occurs, and if this affects venous or lymph-drainage, has not been studied. When the testis or epididymis is sutured to the abdominal wall, it cannot be excluded that this could interfere with either the testicular microcirculation or the secretion of tubule fluid. That the exact position of and temperature increase in the testis are of importance is shown by the observation that the weight of the unilateral, spontaneous ectopic (subcutaneously located) testis is 30 to 37%[21] and the unilateral, spontaneous cryptorchid (inguinal) testis is 23%[22] of that in the corresponding scrotal testis. The temperature increase is approximately 3°C in the ectopic and 5°C in the cryptorchid testis.[21,23,24] When cryptorchidism is induced by fetal estrogen treatment (see below), testis morphology and androgen secretion are markedly different in pararenally and paravesically located abdominal testes.[25,26] Thus, there are several factors that could explain the variability in testicular response in different experimental models. It is likely that the exact position and temperature of the testis must be more carefully defined before data obtained in one model can be directly adapted to another.

B. In Prepubertal Rats

Some investigators have argued that congenitally cryptorchid testes have never been located in the scrotum and have therefore tried to prevent testicular descent before it normally occurs, or at least to reposition the testis shortly after spontaneous descent. In several mammalian species, testicular descent occurs shortly after birth.[1,27] In these species it is thus possible to induce cryptorchidism by preventing descent. In the rat, the cauda epididymides descends into a small scrotal sac soon after birth,[27,29-31] but scrotal development is not complete until about 40 d after birth.[32] Several investigators have induced experimental cryptorchidism in rats between 16 to 25 d of age using the same surgical methods as in adult animals, some with the intent to prevent testicular descent.[13,33-42] This, however, was not achieved since descent actually starts earlier and a temperature difference of 0.7°C is already present between the abdomen and the descending testis in the 16-d-old rat.[43] Thus, in those studies, semidescended testes were returned to the abdomen.

It appears that both closing the inguinal canal or suturing the testis to the abdominal wall in immature rats result in a similar reduction in testis weight, but no systematic comparison of the morphological and functional effects of these two methods on rats is available. The effect on testis weight is, however, apparently greater when cryptorchidism is induced in immature rather than in adult rats using the same method. The unilaterally abdominal testis weighs 14 to 23%,[13,39,44,45] and the bilateral testis 20 to 31%[34,36,38] of controls when experimental cryptorchidism is induced by suturing the inguinal canal in immature rats and when the result is measured at adult age. This observation suggests that the effect of experimental cryptorchidism may be influenced by the age of the animal used. That this is the case was shown by Moore,[28] who found that the effect on testis weight and androgen secretion were clearly dependent on the age of the animal. The effect was more pronounced in immature animals than in adult animals, even when the duration of cryptorchidism was similar. It should be noted that this age-dependent difference was also evident when adult rats of different ages were compared. The older the animal, the less effect on testis weight. Other studies suggest that experimental cryptorchidism induced in immature and adult rats may result in different effects on testis function. Clegg[39] reported a subnormal Leydig cell size in unilaterally abdominal testis when cryptorchidism was induced in 25- to 27-d-old rats, but Risbridger et al.[46] reported an increase in Leydig cell size utilizing adult rats. A similar difference was noted in bilateral cryptorchidism where Clegg[39] observed a normal Leydig cell size whereas Risbridger et al.[46] and Kerr et al.[9] noted a marked Leydig cell hypertrophy using adult rats. A difference between cryptorchidism induced in immature and in adult animals has also been noted in other species. Barenton et al.[47] induced experimental cryptorchidism in immature lambs and in adult rams and observed that the effects on Sertoli and Leydig cells were dependent on the age when cryptorchidism was induced.

C. By Preventing Testicular Descent in Newborn Rats

In 1978, we reported that testicular descent could be prevented in the neonatal rat by cutting the lower part of the gubernaculum testis,[31] and this was later confirmed by others.[48] At birth, the rat testis is lying in the abdominal cavity. The vaginal process has just started to form and the gubernaculum testis is easily identified. By transecting the lower part of the gubernaculum testis, the development of the vaginal process and scrotal sac are prevented and the testis on the operated side remains located in the abdomen. The contralateral testis gradually descends and the scrotum develops. The exact date when testicular descent occurs in rats is difficult to define and this may explain why some investigators claim to have prevented descent in rats up to 35 d of age. If descent is considered to be complete when the cauda epididymis is lying in the bottom of the scrotal sac, it is completed a few days after birth.[27,29,31,49] If descent is considered to be complete only when the testis is lying in the bottom of a fully developed scrotum, then descent does not occur until approximately 40 d of age.[49] The temperature difference between the descending testis and the abdominal cavity is of fundamental importance for testicular development. Using thermocouples, we observed no temperature difference in the 12-d-old rat, but at 16 d of age the descending testis was approximately 0.7°C cooler than the abdominal temperature.[43] This experimental model was named *primary* cryptorchidism[50] to distinguish it from the condition in which descended testes are returned to the abdomen (*secondary* cryptorchidism). Using experimental primary cryptorchid rats, we have examined development, morphology, and function of the abdominal testis using a variety of techniques.

In summary, we observed the first morphological changes in Sertoli cells in some stages of the spermatogenic cycle in the unilateral abdominal testis in the 16-d-old rat.[43] These changes were already apparent when the temperature difference between the two testes was very small, only approximately 0.7°C.[43] The abdominal Sertoli cells contained an increased amount of lipid droplets, but apart from this we did not observe any additional signs of Sertoli cell malfunction at this age.[43] In contrast, tubule lumen formation, which is initiated by Sertoli cell fluid secretion, occurred slightly earlier in the abdominal than in the contralateral scrotal testis, and the abdominal testis weighed slightly more than the scrotal testis at this age[43,54] (Bergh et al. unpublished). A similar, accelerated development in the abdominal testis during the early postnatal period was also noted when cryptorchidism was induced in mice by fetal estrogen treatment.[25] The mechanism behind this early change in Sertoli cell function and the reason why Sertoli cells in some stages of the spermatogenic cycle are more sensitive than others is unknown. This early lipid accumulation is not secondary to germ cell degeneration,[43,51] but hypothetically direct changes in Sertoli cell lipid metabolism, possibly in the cholesterol-ester hydrolase,[52] Hoffman, Bergh, and Olivecrona, unpublished) could be involved. No morphological signs of germ cell dysfunction were observed at this age and Leydig cell morphology and testosterone secretion were apparently unaffected,[53,54] (Bergh et al., unpublished). Four days later, when the temperature difference had increased to 1.5°C, some germ cells, primarily primary spermatocytes lying on the luminal side of the newly formed blood testis barrier, were degenerating, particularly in the same tubular segments in which Sertoli cell malfunction was noted 4 d earlier.[43,49] At this age, additional morphological signs of Sertoli cell malfunction, such as dilatation of the SER and formation of ''vacuoles'' between adjacent Sertoli cells were observed.[43,51] Sertoli cell androgen binding protein (ABP), estrogen, and probably inhibin secretion were also markedly reduced.[54] We suggested that the earliest effect of cryptorchidism occurs in Sertoli cells and that this may later affect adjacent germ cells. Supporting the suggestion that Sertoli cells are directly sensitive to the abdominal milieu is the observation that similar morphological changes also occur at the same time in Sertoli cells in experimental abdominal testes that lack germ cells from birth as a result of fetal irradiation (so-called Sertoli cell-only rats.[51]) Moreover, Hagenäs et al.,[55] who induced secondary cryptorchidism in Sertoli cell only-testes, observed reduced ABP secretion.

Leydig cell morphology is apparently unaffected up to 30 d of age in our experimental model, but, later, Leydig cell size is markedly reduced in the unilateral abdominal testis compared to that in the contralateral scrotal testis[53] and the smooth endoplasmic reticulum is poorly developed.[58] In adult unilaterally cryptorchid rats, the secretion of testosterone into the testicular vein is considerably reduced, both under basal conditions and after human chorionic gonadotropin (hCG) stimulation.[56,57] In vitro studies indicate that this is partially due to an overall reduction steroidogenesis.[58] In addition, a block in steroidogenesis at the 17α hydroxylase and 17—20 lyase steps has been observed both in vivo and in vitro.[58,59] This block may be related to the fourfold increase in testicular estrogen concentration in these abdominal testes.[60,61] The reason for Leydig cell malfunction is not known since Leydig cells are not sensitive to abdominal temperatures per se when studied in vitro.[62] However, tubule damage occurs prior to that in Leydig cells[43] and recent studies have shown that tubules secrete several factors, both inhibitory and stimulatory, which influence the activity of Leydig cells.[63-66] The size of Leydig cells lying close to tubules vary in phase with the spermatogenetic cycle. The largest Leydig cells are observed close to tubules in stages VII to VIII.[67,68] In unilaterally cryptorchid testes, induced in either newborn or adult animals, this stage-dependent variation in Leydig cell size is lost.[68,69] These data clearly suggest that tubule damage induces the Leydig cell dysfunction by disturbing the paracrine interaction between tubules and Leydig cells.

The reduced basal and hCG-stimulated testosterone secretion *in vivo* is, in addition to a direct effect in the Leydig cells, also a secondary effect of insufficient blood flow and vascular permeability in the abdominal testis.[57] Total testicular blood flow, the volume density of interstitial blood vessels, the total endothelial surface area, and vascular permeability are all reduced in the unilaterally primary abdominal rat testis.[56,57] Although the reason for these vascular changes is unknown, it is likely that they could be related to the disturbed Leydig cell and tubule function since Leydig cells and possibly also the tubules are involved in the control of blood flow and vascular permeability in the testis.[63,64,70] The morphology and function of testicular macrophages are also changed in unilateral abdominal testes, possibly secondary to Leydig cell dysfunction.[71] The functional changes in the tubules and interstitium in this experimental model of cryptorchidism are thus rather well characterized.

Testicular descent has also been prevented in rats by suturing the testis to the abdominal wall in immature rats less than 5 d old.[72,73] Although no systematic studies comparing this method with the one in which the gubernaculum has been cut are available, it is likely that the risk of direct testicular damage is greater when the very small testis in neonatal rats is sutured to the abdominal wall, than in the procedure where the gubernaculum is cut but the testes are left untouched. When testes from 3-d-old rats were sutured to the abdominal wall, earlier and more pronounced reductions in testis weight and androgen secretion were seen, particularly in the bilateral abdominal testis,[72] than in the model where the gubernaculum testis was cut.[53,74] Thus, the effect on the testis may be different in these two methods. Whether the greater changes seen in the sutured testes are caused by direct trauma to the testes or if other factors are involved remains to be elucidated.

III. ON DIFFERENCES IN TESTIS MORPHOLOGY AND FUNCTION IN DIFFERENT EXPERIMENTAL MODELS

A. Primary vs. Secondary Experimental Cryptorchidism

Experimental cryptorchidism may thus be induced in two principally different ways, by preventing testicular descent (primary) or by returning descended testes to the abdomen (secondary). The effects on the testis appear to be highly dependent on which of these techniques is used (Table 2), although it cannot be fully excluded that the differences between these models could be related to other factors such as the duration of cryptorchidism.

When testicular descent was prevented in newborn rats, we observed small Leydig cells in the unilateral abdominal testes and a slight hypertrophy (a 13% increase in cell profile area which was not statistically significant) in the adult primary bilateral abdominal testes.[53,71,74] Similarly, Jegou et al.[12] operating on 14-d-old rats, found a slight increase in Leydig cell profile area (15%) in the bilateral abdominal testes. In striking contrast, Leydig cell size was considerably increased both in uni- and bilateral abdominal testes when cryptorchidism was induced in adult rats.[9,46] Moreover, Leydig cell number per testis was decreased in secondary bilateral[76] but unaffected in primary bilateral[71,74] cryptorchidism. The differences between unilaterally abdominal Leydig cells in primary and secondary cryptorchidism is also evident in *in vitro* studies. Testosterone secretion *in vitro* was subnormal in primary,[58,72] but supranormal in secondary, unilateral cryptorchidism.[46] It should be noted that Leydig cell size was reduced in the unilateral congenitally cryptorchid testis in rats, dogs, cats, horses, pigs, goats, and humans,[77-81] and, in congenitally maldescended rat testes, steroidogenesis was decreased *in vitro*.[21]

Vascular permeability and blood flow regulation are disturbed in the primary unilateral abdominal rat testes.[56,57] Whether similar vascular changes are present in secondary cryptorchidism is less well established, although vascular permeability is subnormal in bilateral

Table 2

COMPARISON BETWEEN TESTES IN ADULT PRIMARY AND SECONDARY UNILATERAL CRYPTORCHID RATS IN RELATION TO THAT IN THE CONTRALATERAL SCROTAL TESTIS

Parameter measured	Primary	Ref.	Secondary	Ref.
Leydig cell size	Decreased	53	Increased	46
Leydig cell number/testis	Normal	53, 85	Not studied	
Testis testosterone concentration	Decreased	53, 72	Decreased	140
IF testosterone concentration	Decreased	57	Decreased	15
Testosterone secretion *in vitro*	Decreased	58, 72	Increased	46
LH receptors/testis	Decreased	85	Decreased	46
LHRH receptors/testis	Normal	85	Not studied	
Estrogen receptors/testis	Normal	60, 85	Normal	140
IF volume				
Basal	Decreased	57	Normal	15
			Increased	82
After hCG	Increased over basal	57	Unaffected compared to basal	82
Blood flow (ml/g testis)				
Basal	Increased	56	Normal	83
After hCG	Almost unaffected compared to basal	57	Not studied	
Volume density of blood vessels in the interstitium	Decreased	57	Not studied	
Sertoli cell protein secretion	Decreased	54	Decreased	55
Sertoli cell number/testis	Normal	85	Not studied	
FSH receptors/testis	Decreased	85	Decreased	46
Size of testicular macrophages	Decreased	71	Not studied	

secondary cryptorchidism.[14] When a mature testis is returned to the abdomen, it contains a vasculature developed to support a large tubular mass. To what extent these blood vessels are influenced by secondary cryptorchidism is not known. In primary cryptorchidism, the vasculature is probably developed only to support a very small testis. It is, therefore, not surprising if differences in blood flow and vascular permeability exist between primary and secondary cryptorchidism, and indirect evidence suggests that this is probably the case. Interstitial fluid (IF) volume is reduced in unilateral primary abdominal testes,[57] but normal or increased in unilateral secondary cryptorchidism.[15,82] Moreover, hCG treatment increases IF volume in primary,[57] but not in secondary, unilaterally abdominal testes.[82] Testicular blood flow (milliliters per gram of testis) is comparable to that in a scrotal testis in secondary unilateral cryptorchidism,[83] but increased in primary cryptorchidism.[56] We recently observed that intratesticular pressure is increased up to 40 mmHg in the abdominal testes of experimentally primary unilaterally cryptorchid rats 24 h after stimulation with hCG, and that this is probably caused by a marked increase in vascular permeability and insufficient lymph drainage.[84] In secondary cryptorchid adult rats this increase in pressure was considerably less pronounced.[84] In conclusion, the effect of experimental cryptorchidism on the interstitial tissue is highly different in primary and secondary experimental cryptorchidism.

It is, however, likely (but not proven) that the differences between primary and secondary cryptorchidism is smaller in the tubules than in the interstitium. Obviously, the short-term tubular effects are different in these two approaches since tubules of different morphologies are affected, and the early signs of accelerated Sertoli cell function in primary cryptorchidism[43] (Bergh et al., unpublished) have not been observed in secondary cryptorchidism. However, the morphological and functional changes in Sertoli cells, i.e., dilatation of the SER, lipid accumulation, and the appearance of vacuoles between adjacent Sertoli cells, occur in both models,[10,43,51] and in both models Sertoli cells in some tubular stages appear to be more susceptible than others.[69] Similar reductions in follicle stimulating hormone (FSH)-receptors and protein secretion have been described in both models.[11,54,59,75,85]

It is not surprising that differences exist between the testes in primary and secondary cryptorchidism. The morphological and functional changes in an abdominal testis are probably caused by primary changes in temperature-sensitive cells (possibly in the Sertoli cells), but also by secondary changes caused by tubule malfunction.[68,86] These changes could be caused by alterations in the local paracrine mechanisms operating between the tubules and interstitial tissue.[63,64] The observation that the most pronounced differences between primary and secondary abdominal testes are noted in the interstitium suggest that these paracrine mechanisms are affected differently when cryptorchidism is induced in immature, rather than in adult, animals. For several reasons this is not surprising. Sertoli cell function is clearly different in immature and adult animals.[87,88] In primary cryptorchidism, it appears that the earliest changes in the abdominal tubules take place in Sertoli cells,[43,51] but in secondary cryptorchidism most investigators claim that the earliest changes occur in developed germ cells (see below). Sertoli cell function is in part controlled by germ cells. Some types of germ cells have stimulatory effects whereas others probably have inhibitory effects.[65,87,89-91] Therefore, it is likely that the types of germ cells degenerating is obviously different in primary and secondary cryptorchidism, and this may influence Sertoli cell function differently. Moreover, the first wave of spermatogenesis is probably regulated differently than the following ones, and it is less susceptible to abdominal temperatures.[92] Against this background it is not surprising that the secondary changes, occurring in non-temperature-sensitive cells, are different in primary and secondary cryptorchidism.

B. Bilateral vs. Unilateral Cryptorchidism

Unfortunately, only a few studies have been designed to compare uni- and bilateral cryptorchidism. Such studies may give important information on the pathophysiology of cryptorchidism, particularly for the understanding of the secondary changes induced in nontemperature-sensitive cells. Most investigators, irrespective of experimental model and species, have noted that the weight of the bilateral abdominal testis is larger than that of the unilateral abdominal testis. Bilateral cryptorchidism in rats results in markedly increased levels of FSH and luteinizing hormone (LH), however, on the other hand most investigators claim gonadotropins to be unaffected by unilateral cryptorchidism.[37,93,94] Sharpe et al.,[95] however, found an increase in FSH and Risbridger et al.[46] observed a temporary increase in LH. The differences in testis weight have, therefore, been assumed to be related to differences in gonadotropin stimulation. Clegg[39] observed that spermatogenesis was slightly less damaged in bi- than in unilateral abdominal testes. Bergh and Damber,[74] by preventing testicular descent, observed that the total tubule length was larger in bi- than in unilaterally cryptorchid testes, but that the degree of damage to the spermatogenic epithelium was similar. The size of bilateral abdominal Leydig cells is larger than that in unilateral abdominal Leydig cells both in experimental primary and secondary cryptorchidism.[46,74] Testicular testosterone and estrogen concentrations are lower in uni- than in bilateral primary cryptorchidism.[53,61] Moreover, basal and hCG/LH-stimulated testosterone secretion *in vitro* are also greater in bi- than in unilateral secondary cryptorchidism.[46,96] IF volume and the concentration of testosterone in the interstitial fluid are larger in bi- than in unilateral secondary cryptorchid testes.[15] These data clearly suggest that Leydig cell function is better preserved in bi- than in unilateral abdominal testes. The secretion of testosterone from bilateral secondary cryptorchid testes *in vivo*, both basally and after stimulation with a low dose of hCG, is however, lower than in normal testes.[9,11,97] This suggests that the increased gonadotropin stimulation in bilateral cryptorchidism may improve Leydig cell function in comparison with that in unilateral abdominal testes, but the function is not fully normalized *in vivo* (testosterone secretion *in vitro* is, however, supranormal[46,86]). These differences in Leydig cell function in bi- and unilateral abdominal testes clearly indicate that Leydig cell function in cryptorchidism is not a direct reflection of the supranormal temperature per se, but that compensatory changes in gonadotropins and in local paracrine mechanisms are more important.

Unfortunately, Sertoli cell function in bi- and unilateral abdominal testes has not been compared, thus, the extent to which cryptorchidism-induced Sertoli cell malfunction (probably a keystone for the understanding of the pathophysiology of cryptorchidism) can be affected by hormonal stimulation and changes in the local paracrine milieu in the testis cannot be evaluated. Indirect evidence does, however, suggest that abdominal Sertoli cells respond to hormonal stimulation, since total tubule length and the total number of germ cells per testis are larger in bi- than in unilateral abdominal testes.[39,74] That abdominal Sertoli cells may respond to gonadotrophin stimulation is also shown by the transient normalization of FSH receptor numbers in the unilateral abdominal testis after hCG treatment.[59] The seminiferous tubules secrete a factor which stimulates Leydig cells *in vitro,* particularly in testes with tubule damage. The secretion of this factor was lower in bi- than in unilateral cryptorchidism, suggesting differences in tubule protein secretion in bi- and unilateral abdominal testes.[15]

Other aspects of testis function have not been compared in uni- and bilateral cryptorchid testes. For example, all data on basal and hCG-stimulated blood flow and vascular permeability in primary experimental cryptorchidism have been obtained in unilateral cryptorchidism.[56,57] In secondary cryptorchidism, most studies deal with bilateral cryptorchidism.[14] Nevertheless, it is likely that vascular permeability is different in bi- compared to unilateral secondary cryptorchidism, since IF volume is larger in bi- than in unilateral abdominal testes.[15] This difference is not surprising since vascular permeability in the testis is probably controlled by Leydig cells and tubules[63,64,70] and both have different functions in bi- and unilateral cryptorchidism.

The morphology of testicular macrophages is less influenced in bi- than in unilateral abdominal testes.[71] The reason for this is unknown, but the functional activity of Leydig cells and macrophages is in some way correlated, and the difference in macrophage morphology between bi- and unilateral primary abdominal testes may thus be related to the difference in Leydig cell function.

It is evident that morphology and cell function differ between bi- and unilateral abdominal testes (summarized in Table 3) and, thus, data obtained in one of these types of cryptorchidism cannot be directly applied to the other, particularly when different experimental methods are used.

C. Effect of Duration

Obviously the duration of cryptorchidism may also explain differences in the effects on the testis in different studies of experimental cryptorchidism (see also Section II.B). After experimental cryptorchidism in adult animals, the tubules start to degenerate immediately, and, after some time, changes are also noted in the interstitial tissue. These changes occur during the first 3 to 4 weeks, but after this time testis morphology and weight are stabilized.[9-11,75,97,98] Thus, the exact duration of experimental cryptorchidism is important when examining testes that have been cryptorchid for less than 1 month. It is generally assumed that the condition is fairly stable thereafter. However, apart from the relatively stable weight, this may not be the case. Lloyd[99] induced bilateral cryptorchidism at 1.5 months of age and followed the animals up to 13.5 months. He found that testosterone secretion was increased at 3 months, normal at 4.5 months, and reduced from 7.5 months. This finding clearly indicates that the exact duration of cryptorchidism may also be of importance when comparing different studies describing the long-term effects of cryptorchidism.

Table 3
**COMPARISON BETWEEN BI- AND UNILATERAL ABDOMINAL
TESTES IN ADULT RATS**

Parameter measured	Results	Ref.
Serum concentration of FSH and LH	Bi > uni	93
Testis weight	Bi > uni	15, 74
Leydig cell size	Bi > uni	46, 74
Number of Leydig cells/testis	Bi = uni	74
	Bi > uni	39
LH receptors/testis	Bi > uni	46
Testis testosterone concentration (basal and after LH)	Bi > uni	61, 74
IF testosterone concentration	Bi > uni	15
Testosterone secretion *in vitro* (basal and after LH)	Bi > uni	96
Testicular estrogen concentration	Bi > uni	61
IF volume	Bi > uni	15
Blood flow	Not compared	
Sertoli cell morphology	Not compared	
Number of Sertoli cells/testis	Bi > uni	39
Sertoli cell protein secretion	Not compared	
FSH receptors/testis	Bi > uni	46
Total tubule length	Bi > uni	74
Tubule diameter	Bi = uni	74
Development of spermatogenesis	Bi > uni	39
	Bi = uni	74
Size of testicular macrophages	Bi > uni	71

D. Species Differences

Surgical induction of cryptorchidism shortly after birth has also been induced in other species. For example, Antliff and Young[100] and Atkinson[101] rendered guinea pigs surgically cryptorchid within 1 week after birth, and Skinner and Rowson[102] did likewise to immature lambs and calves. Unfortunately, too little is known of the morphology and function in congenitally cryptorchid guinea pigs, lambs, and calves to evaluate how close these experimental models mimic congenital cryptorchidism in these species. Experimental cryptorchidism has also been induced at birth in pigs and this will be discussed below.

Experimental cryptorchidism has also been obtained by returning descended testes to the abdomen in several species. Although the results will not be discussed here, it appears that the general effects of cryptorchidism are similar in most species. However, some important differences have been noted in different species. When unilateral cryptorchidism is induced, the scrotal testis is either unaffected or slightly hypertrophic in most species.[45,49,102,103] When dogs are used, degenerative changes are noted in the scrotal testis, changes that are probably caused by autoimmune mechanisms.[104-107] Antibodies formed against germ cells in the abdominal testes later also attack the scrotal testis, but this phenomenon has only been described in experimentally cryptorchid dogs.

IV. CONGENITAL VS. EXPERIMENTAL SURGICAL CRYPTORCHIDISM

When comparing experimental models of cryptorchidism, one important factor is to evaluate how closely they mimic the congenital condition and to what extent they can be used to elucidate the pathophysiology of the human cryptorchid testis.

A. Congenital vs. Experimental Cryptorchidism in Rats

There are strains of rats in which spontaneous maldescent (most often unilateral) is occasionally observed. In some,[21,23] the testis is located subcutaneously in an ectopic position in the inguinal region. In others, the testis is lying in the cranial part of the inguinal canal.[22,108,109] It is likely that spontaneous ectopic and cryptorchid testes are not identical (see above), but no direct comparison between those two types of maldescended testes have been published (testis morphology is, however, different in human ectopic and cryptorchid testes[110]). Obviously, a detailed comparison between testicular function in spontaneous cryptorchidism with that in various experimental models of cryptorchidism would be most interesting and could solve the question of whether the spontaneous cryptorchid gonad is damaged from the start or whether all morphological and functional changes can be mimicked in the experimental condition. Such comparisons are important for the characterization of an experimental model.

Hellbach[22] and Krausse,[109] studying congenitally cryptorchid rats, observed germ cell degeneration and a later occurring thickening of the tubule wall. These changes appear similar and occur at the same age as those in the experimental model.[43,49] In both congenital and experimental primary cryptorchid testes, the first wave of spermatogenesis seems to be less susceptible to cryptorchidism than subsequent waves.[22,49] Numerous degenerating primary spermatocytes are observed after 20 d of age, nevertheless at 30 d of age occasional round spermatids are observed. They later disappear and are not observed in the subsequent cycles. That the first wave of spermatogenesis is less susceptible to abdominal temperature than later waves has also been shown by transplanting neonatal rat testes into the abdominal testis of an adult rat.[92] Unfortunately, neither Sertoli cell morphology and function nor Leydig cell function has been analyzed in congenitally cryptorchid rats. However, Leydig cell size is reduced similarly in the congenital and experimental condition and this change occurs after the tubule damage.[22,53] In the congenitally ectopic rat testis, the Leydig cells have an immature morphology and secrete subnormal amounts of testosterone in vitro,[21] comparable to our experimental model.[53,54,59,85] Sertoli cell secretion of ABP is reduced in both ectopic[23] and experimentally primary abdominal rat testes.[54] The number of blood vessels in the interstitium is reduced in the ectopic testis and permeability is probably also reduced,[21] thus the vascular changes are similar to those seen in the experimental model.[56,57]

Unfortunately, other aspects of morphology and function have not been studied in these congenitally maldescended rat testes making it impossible to evaluate how close experimental primary cryptorchidism mimics congenital maldescent. However, in the data currently available, no obvious differences between our model and the congenital condition have been noted. Experimental primary cryptorchidism, in contrast to secondary cryptorchidism, may thus be a valid model for congenital cryptorchidism in rats.

B. Experimental Cryptorchidism in Rats as a Model for Human Cryptorchidism

Most of our current knowledge on testis physiology is derived from studies in rats. Thus, a good experimental model for cryptorchidism in rats would be of some importance. Rat models may, however, be inadequate when trying to understand the pathophysiology of cryptorchidism in humans. It is obvious that reintroduction of a descended, more or less mature, rat testis into the abdomen does not mimic the congenital condition where the testis has never been located in the scrotum. Such rat testes contain cell types that are not present in the testes of cryptorchid infants, and the cell types present are not in the same functional and developmental stage. By returning mature testes to the abdominal cavity, it has been shown that primary spermatocytes and round spermatids are particularly sensitive to abdominal temperatures,[5,111-114] possibly because their cellular membranes are unstable at abdominal temperatures[115] and protein synthesis in round spermatids is negatively influenced by abdominal temperatures.[116-118] This information is, however, of limited value when trying to understand the early tubular and Leydig cell changes in congenitally cryptorchid human and pig testes. In these species, the tubules contain only undeveloped Sertoli cells and gonocytes at the age when morphological changes are observed in the cryptorchid testes. Leydig cell atrophy was noted in 1-year-old cryptorchid boys[80] and a reduced number of germ cells was noted in 1-year-old[119] or in 2-year-old boys.[80,120] In congenitally cryptorchid pigs, Leydig cell atrophy is observed the 2nd week of life and the number of germ cells is reduced shortly thereafter.[78,79] These changes are not present at birth suggesting that they are induced by the malposition, and they can be fully mimicked by inducing experimental cryptorchidism in normal pigs at birth.[121] In experimental and congenital cryptorchidism in rats, it is clear that the tubular changes preceded those in Leydig cells, but this relation is not evident in congenital cryptorchidism in pigs and humans. Whether the early Leydig cell dysfunction in these testes is caused by the tubule malfunction, as in experimental cryptorchidism in rats, is thus uncertain.

The principal disadvantage with the rat model in which testicular descent is prevented is that spermatogenesis already starts at birth in this species. At the time when a temperature difference is established between the testis and the abdomen, testis morphology in the rat is different from that in the newborn humans and other species in which spermatogenesis does not start until puberty (in the 12- to 16-d-old rat the tubules contain maturing Sertoli cells, different types of spermatogonia, and primary spermatocytes up to the pachytene level). These immature rat testes thus contain cell types either not present or at a developmental stage different from that in the immature cryptorchid testis in humans and pigs. Thus, the same objections raised against secondary cryptorchidism are also relevant here. The observation in our model that maturing Sertoli cells are particularly sensitive to abdominal temperatures in prepubertal rats may thus not necessarily explain the tubular damage in human cryptorchid testes. On the other hand, that the early germ cell degeneration in human cryptorchidism is caused by Sertoli cell malfunction as in rats, cannot be excluded. Unfortunately, Sertoli cell function has not been studied in cryptorchid testes in humans and pigs and, until this is done the extent to which experimental primary cryptorchidism in rats may be used to elucidate the pathophysiology of the early tubule damage in human cryptorchidism cannot be evaluated. However, Sertoli cells in 2-year-old cryptorchid boys have a vacuolated cytoplasm and the space between adjacent Sertoli cells is often dilated,[120] changes which are very similar to those occurring early in the rat model.[43,51] However, in striking contrast to the rat model, Sertoli cell lipid accumulation was not noted in human cryptorchidism.[80,120] Our rat model is also complicated by the fact that immature rats are poikiolothermic.[122] Rats are not able to maintain a body temperature of 37°C until at about 17 d of age. Thus, the average abdominal temperature is increasing during development, whereas it is probably constant in the human.

V. EXPERIMENTAL CRYPTORCHIDISM IN OTHER SPECIES AS A MODEL FOR HUMAN CRYPTORCHIDISM

It can, thus, be questioned whether the pathophysiological changes occurring in the cryptorchid human testis can be elucidated by returning descended testes to the abdomen or by preventing testicular descent in the rat. A more appropriate model for the early functional changes in human cryptorchid testes should probably be sought in a species in which spermatogenesis does not start until puberty. The important observation by van Straaten[121] that all morphological changes noted in the congenital unilaterally cryptorchid pig testis can be mimicked by inducing experimental cryptorchidism at birth in that species is thus most interesting. However, early occurring morphological changes have also been described in the scrotal testis in some, but not all, unilaterally cryptorchid boys (e.g., reduced number of gonocytes[119]), but changes in the scrotal testes are not observed in congenitally or experimental cryptorchid pigs.[78,79,121] The pig may thus not be an ideal model for human cryptorchidism. On the other hand, a reduced number of germ cells was not observed in all cryptorchid boys, and it is likely that cryptorchidism in humans may be caused by different mechanisms.[123] There are probably two principally different types of human cryptorchidism: nondescent due to an inherent imperfection in the gonad, or nondescent due to extratesticular factors. It should also be noted that in most patients with cryptorchidism the testis is lying in the inguinal canal or high in the scrotum and more infrequently in the abdomen.[124,125] It is, thus, obvious that a single experimental model cannot mimic all variants of human cryptorchidism. In experimentally cryptorchid dogs, changes are noted in the scrotal testis, but it is doubtful whether the early scrotal changes in humans could be caused by the same mechanisms as in these dogs (see above), since, at this age, no blood-testis barrier is present and the undeveloped germ cells present in these human testes are probably not antigenic. It thus remains to be elucidated whether experimental cryptorchidism in dogs would serve as a model for human cryptorchidism and studies comparing experimental with congenital cryptorchidism in that species are not available.

VI. HORMONALLY INDUCED EXPERIMENTAL CRYPTORCHIDISM

Experimental cryptorchidism may, apart from the surgical methods discussed above, also be induced by treatment of pregnant mice and rats with a single injection of estradiol. This results in unilateral or, more commonly, bilateral cryptorchidism in the male off-spring.[25,80,126-128] The testes are located in variable positions from the abdominal cavity to the lower part of the inguinal canal.[25,26,127] Estrogen-induced cryptorchidism has been explained by inhibition of testicular hormone secretion resulting in a maldevelopment of the gubernaculum and, thus, impaired descent.[126] These animals do, however, show other signs of disturbed development of the sex organs, such as hypospadia and retention of Mullerian-derived organs.[25,26,126-128] Advocates of this model claim that it mimics the congenital condition by disturbing the hypothalamic-hypophysial-testis axis in the fetus and that cryptorchidism in humans is caused by similar mechanisms.[80,125] Estrogen-induced nondescent can be prevented by simultaneous hCG treatment.[80] Moreover, there are epidemiological data linking a fetal excess of estrogen with cryptorchidism,[129-131] but others have not found this connection.[132] If it can be proved that spontaneous cryptorchidism is related to a fetal excess of estrogen, this model is clearly of value. However, if this is not the case, this model is probably inferior to others, since estrogen treatment may have direct effects on the development of the testis and the central nervous system.[133-136] It will thus be difficult to determine which effects on the cryptorchid testis are related to the malposition itself and which are related to other effects of estrogen. Most data on hormonally induced cryptorchidism have been obtained in mice,[25,26,80,127] but there are no studies directly comparing testicular morphology and function in hormonally and surgically induced cryptorchidism in that species. There are, however, probably some principal differences between this model and surgical cryptorchidism. In estrogen-induced cryptorchidism in mice, Leydig cells in the abdominal testis are atrophic at birth.[80] This is not the case in congenital or experimental primary cryptorchidism in rats or in congenital cryptorchidism in pigs (see above). However, in cryptorchid human infants, Leydig cells are reported to be atrophic as in the estrogen model.[80,125] Moreover, in estrogen-induced cryptorchidism, some of the retained testes are located in the abdomen near the bladder, but surprisingly active spermatogenesis can be found in these testes.[25] However, spermatogenesis was not noted if the testis was lying near the kidney.[25] When surgical experimental cryptorchidism is induced by placing the mouse testis in the lower abdomen, no spermatogenesis is seen.[137] The value of hormonally induced cryptorchidism as a model for congenital cryptorchidism can thus be questioned. Moreover, as mentioned previously, all changes noted in the congenitally cryptorchid pig or rat testis can be mimicked by surgical cryptorchidism in these species, suggesting that the malfunction in an abdominal testis may be the result of the malposition itself and not caused by additional hormonal effects on the gonad. However, the value of estrogen-induced cryptorchidism as a model for human cryptorchidism cannot be evaluated properly before more is known about the etiology of human cryptorchidism, particularly the role of estrogen. Indeed, apart from the early Leydig cell atrophy, there are some interesting similarities between this model and human cryptorchidism. In both types, spontaneous descent is noted after birth in some cases,[25] but the mechanism behind this is presently unknown.

VII. SUMMARY

Experimental cryptorchidism may be induced in several ways and the effects on testicular morphology and function are in some respects similar in all models, but in other respects highly different. For example, the function of the abdominal testis is dependent on whether cryptorchidism is induced by preventing testicular descent or by returning descended testes to the abdomen and also whether it is bilateral or unilateral. The species, the age of the animal, and the duration of cryptorchidism are also of importance. Differences in the experimental design may explain some of the contradictory findings reported in different studies.

In contrast to the experimental methods where descended testes are returned to the abdomen, it is probably possible to mimic congenital cryptorchidism in pigs and rats fairly well by inducing surgical cryptorchidism at birth in these species. However, it remains to be shown whether the data obtained in these animal models will be of relevance for the understanding of the pathophysiological changes occurring in human cryptorchidism.

ACKNOWLEDGMENTS

This work was supported by grants from the Swedish Medical Research Council (project number 5935) and the Maud and Birger Gustavsson Foundation.

REFERENCES

1. **Wensing, C. J. G.**, Testicular descent in some domestic mammals. I. Anatomical aspect of testicular descent, *Proc. Kon. Nederl. Akad. Wet.*, 71, 423, 1968.
2. **Shapiro, G. R. and Bodai, B. J.**, Current concepts of the undescended testis, *Surg. Gynecol. Obstet.*, 147, 617, 1978.
3. **Hutson, J. M. and Donahoe, P. K.**, The hormonal control of testicular descent, *Endocr. Rev.*, 7, 270, 1986.
4. **Chilvers, C., Pike, M. C., Forman, D., Fogelman, K., and Wadsworth, M. E. J.**, Apparent doubling of frequency of undescended testis in England and Wales in 1962 to 81, *Lancet*, 1, 330, 1985.
5. **Van Demark, N. L. and Free, M. J.**, Temperature effects, in *The Testis*, Vol. 3, Johnson, A. D., Gomes, W. R., and Van Demark, N. L., Eds., Academic Press, New York, 233 1970.
6. **Cowles, R. B.**, Hypertomia, aspermia, mutation rates and evolution, *Q. Rev. Biol.*, 40, 341, 1965.
7. **Bedford, J. M., Berrios, M., and Dryden, G. L.**, Biology of the scrotum. IV. Testis location and temperature sensitivity, *J. Exp. Zool.*, 224, 379, 1982.
8. **Griffiths, J.**, The structural changes in the testicle of the dog when it is replaced within the abdominal cavity, *J. Anat. London*, 27, 483, 1893.
9. **Kerr, J. B., Rich, K. A., and de Kretser, D. M.**, Alterations of the fine structure and androgen secretion of the interstitial cells in the experimental cryptorchid rat testis, *Biol Reprod.*, 20, 409, 1979.
10. **Kerr, J. B., Rich, K. A., and de Kretser, D. M.**, Effects of experimental cryptorchidism on the ultrastructure and function of the Sertoli cell and peritubular tissue of the rat testis, *Biol. Reprod.*, 21, 823, 1979.
11. **Jegou, B., Risbridger, G. P., and de Kretser, D. M.**, Effects of experimental cryptorchidism on testicular function in adult rats, *J. Androl.*, 4, 88, 1983.

12. **Jégou, B., Peake, R. A., Irby, D. C., and de Kretser, D. M.**, Effects of the induction of experimental cryptorchidism and subsequent orchidopexy on testicular function in immature rats, *Biol. Reprod.*, 30, 179, 1984.

13. **Jahnsen, T., Karpe, B., Attramadal, H., Ritzéen, M., and Hansson, V.**, Changes in isoproterenol-stimulated adenylate cyclase activity in rat testicular tissue during cryptorchidism and after orchidopexy, *J. Reprod. Fertil.*, 70, 443, 1984.

14. **Sharpe, R. M.**, Impaired gonadotrophin uptake in vivo by the cryptorchid rat testis, *J. Reprod. Fertil.*, 67, 379, 1983.

15. **Sharpe, R. M., Kerr, J. B., Fraser, H. M., and Bartlett, J. M. S.**, Intratesticular factors and testosterone secretion, *J. Androl.*, 7, 180, 1986.

16. **Urry, R. L., Dougherty, K. A., and Cockett, A. T.**, Time-dependent alterations in testicular function after experimental cryptorchism, *Surg. Forum*, 26, 574, 1975.

17. **Moore, C. R. and Quick, W. J.**, The scrotum as a temperature regulator for the testes, *Am. J. Physiol.*, 68, 70, 1924.

18. **Grinsted, J., Blendstrup, K., Andreasen, M. P., and Byskov, A. G.**, Temperature measurements of rabbit antral follicles, *J. Reprod. Fertil.*, 60, 149, 1980.

19. **Clegg, E. J.**, Studies on artificial cryptorchidism: degenerative and regenerative changes in the germinal epithelium of the rat testis, *J. Endocrinol.*, 27, 241, 1963.

20. **Gunn, S., Gould, T. C., and Anderson, W. A. D.**, Seasonal variations in endocrine response to cryptorchidism, *Acta Endocrinol.*, 37, 589, 1961.

21. **Chung, K. W., Dressler, J. B., Halterman, M. W., and Allison, J. E.**, Structural and functional abnormality of ectopic testes in rats, *Life Sci.*, 34, 1953, 1984.

22. **Hellbach, G.**, Histometrische untersuchungen an testes von ratten mit hereditär bedingter unilateralen descenssustörungen, Inaugural Dissertation, Frankfurt a.M., 1970.

23. **Dressler, J. B., Allison, J. E., and Chung, K. W.**, Ectopic testes. A heritable mutation in the King-Holzman rat: androgen binding protein in testes and epididymides, *Biol. Reprod.*, 29, 1313, 1983.

24. **Chan, W.-Y., Bates, J. M., Chung, K. W., and Rennert, O. M.**, Abnormal zinc metabolism in unilateral maldescended testes of a mutant rat strain (42379), *Proc. Soc. Exp. Biol. Med.*, 182, 549, 1986.

25. **Jean, C.**, Croissance et structure des testicules cryptorchides chez les souris nées de méres traitées a l'oestradiol pendant la gestation, *Ann. Endocrinol.*, 34, 669, 1973.

26. **Jean, C., André, M., Jean, C., Berger, M., De Turckheim, M., and Veyssiére, G.**, Estimation of testosterone and androstenedione in the plasma and testes of cryptorchid offspring of mice treated with oestradiol during pregnancy, *J. Reprod. Fertil.*, 44, 235, 1975.

27. **Wensing, C. J. G.**, Testicular descent in the rat and a comparison of this process in the rat with that in the pig, *Anat. Record.*, 214, 154, 1986.

28. **Moore, C. R.**, Hormone secretion by experimental cryptorchid testes, *Yale J. Biol. Med.*, 203, 1944.

29. **Backhouse, K. M.**, The cremaster muscle and testicular descent in the rat, *J. Physiol. (London)*, 151, 41, 1960.

30. **Backhouse, K. M.**, Development and descent of the testis, *Eur. J. Pediatr.*, 139, 249, 1982.

31. **Bergh, A., Helander, H. F., and Wahlqvist, L.**, Studies on factors governing testicular descent in the rat — particularly the role of gubernaculum testis, *Int. J. Androl.*, 1, 342, 1978.

32. **Green, E. C.**, The rat in laboratory investigation, Farris, E. J. and Griffith, J. Q., Eds., Lippincott, Philadelphia, 1949.

33. **Karpe, B., Plöen, L., Hagenäs, L., and Ritzéen, E. M.**, Recovery of testicular functions after surgical treatment of experimental cryptorchidism in the rat, *Int. J. Androl.*, 4, 145, 1981.

34. **Karpe, B., Plöen, L., and Ritzén, E. M.**, Maturation of the juvenile rat testis after surgical treatment of cryptorchidism, *J. Androl.*, 7, 154, 1984.

35. **Davis, J. R. and Firlit, C. F.**, The germinal epithelium of cryptorchid testes experimentally induced in prepubertal and adult rats, *Fertil. Steril.*, 17, 187, 1966.

36. **Ojeda, S. R., Jameson, H. E., and McCann, S. M.**, Plasma prolactin levels in maturing intact and cryptorchid male rats: development of stress response, *Soc. Exp. Biol. Med.*, 151, 310, 1976.

37. **Swerdloff, R. S., Walsh, P. C., Jacobs, H. S., and Odell, W. D.**, Serum LH and FSH during sexual maturation in the male rat: effect of castration and cryptorchidism, *Endocrinology*, 88, 120, 1970.

38. **Dierickx, P. and Verhoeven, G.**, Effect of different methods of germinal cell destruction on rat testis, *J. Reprod. Fertil.*, 59, 5, 1980.

39. **Clegg, E. J.**, Studies on artificial cryptorchidism, the histological appearances of unilateral and bilateral abdominal testes in the rat, *J. Endocrinol.*, 33, 269, 1965.

40. **Heindel, J. J., Berkowitz, A., Steinberger, A., and Strada, S. J.**, Modification of Sertoli cell responsiveness to FSH by cryptorchidism and hypophysectomy in immature and adult rats, *J. Androl.*, 3, 337, 1982.

41. **Cedenho, A. P., Hayashi, H., and Sadi, A.**, Fertilizing capacity of early pubertal cryptorchid rat after orchiopexy, *Arch. Androl.*, 10, 269, 1983.

42. **Grizard, G., Boucher, D., Andre, M., and Jarrige, J. F.,** Evolutions des gonadotropines et de la testostérone plasmatiques et des récepteurs tecticulaires a la lutropine chez le rat normal et cryptorchide, *Reprod. Nutr. Dév.,* 20, 261, 1980.

43. **Bergh, A.,** Early morphological changes in the abdominal testes in immature unilaterally cryptorchid rats, *Int. J. Androl.,* 6, 73, 1983.

44. **Hochberg, Z., Amit, T., Youdim, M. B., Bar-Maor, H., and Jehuda, A.,** Prolactin binding by testes of unilaterally cryptorchid rats: the effect of hCG, testosterone, prolactin and orchiopexy, *Acta Endocrinol.,* 102, 144, 1983.

45. **Clegg, E. J.,** Studies on artificial cryptorchidism. Compensatory changes in the scrotal testes of unilaterally cryptorchid rats, *J. Endocrinol.,* 33, 259, 1965.

46. **Risbridger, G. P., Kerr, J. B., and de Kretser, D. M.,** Evaluation of Leydig cell function and gonadotropin binding in unilateral and bilateral cryptorchidism: evidence for local control of Leydig cell function by the seminiferous tubule, *Biol. Reprod.,* 24, 534, 1981.

47. **Barenton, B., Blanc, M. R., Caraty, A., Hochereau-de Reviers, M. T., Perreau, C., and Saumande, J.,** Effect of cryptorchidism in the ram: changes in the concentrations of testosterone and estradiol and receptors for LH and FSH in the testis, and its histology, *Mol. Cell. Endocrinol.,* 28, 13, 1982.

48. **Frey, H. L. and Rajfer, J.,** Role of the gubernaculum and intraabdominal pressure in the process of testicular descent, *J. Urol.,* 131, 574, 1984.

49. **Bergh, A. and Helander, H. F.,** Testicular development in the unilaterally cryptorchid rat, *Int. J. Androl.,* 1, 440, 1978.

50. **Bergh, A.,** Studies on Experimental Primary Cryptorchidism in Rats, Thesis, Umeå University Medical Dissertations, 44, 1979.

51. **Bergh, A.,** Morphological signs of a direct effect of experimental cryptorchidism on the Sertoli cells in rats irradiated as fetuses, *Biol. Reprod.,* 24, 145, 1981.

52. **Durham, L. A. and Grogan, W. M.,** Characterization of multiple forms of cholesteryl ester hydrolase in the rat testis, *J. Biol. Chem.,* 259, 7433, 1984.

53. **Bergh, A. and Damber, J.-E.,** Morphometric and functional investigation on the Leydig cells in experimental unilateral cryptorchidism in the rat, *Int. J. Androl.,* 1, 549, 1978.

54. **Bergh, A., Damber, J.-E., and Ritzén, E. M.,** Early signs of Sertoli and Leydig cell dysfunction in the abdominal testes of immature unilaterally cryptorchid rats, *Int. J. Androl.,* 7, 398, 1984.

55. **Hagenäs, L., Ritzén, E. M., Svensson, J., and Hansson, V.,** Temperature dependence of Sertoli cell function, *Int. J. Androl.,* 2, 449, 1978.

56. **Damber, J.-E., Bergh, A., and Janson, P.-O.,** Testicular blood flow and testosterone concentration in the spermatic venous blood in rats with experimental cryptorchidism, *Acta Endocrinol.,* 88, 611, 1978.

57. **Damber, J.-E., Bergh, A., and Daehlin, L.,** Testicular blood flow, vascular permeability and testosterone production after hCG stimulation in adult unilaterally cryptorchid rats, *Endocrinology,* 117, 1906, 1985.

58. **Bergh, A., Berg, A. Å., Damber, J.-E., Hammar, M., and Selstam, G.,** Steroid biosynthesis and Leydig cell morphology in adult unilaterally cryptorchid rats, *Acta Endocrinol.,* 107, 556, 1984.

59. **Huhtaniemi, I., Bergh, A., Nikula, H., and Damber, J.-E.,** Differences in the regulation of steroidogenesis and tropic hormone receptors between the scrotal and abdominal testes of unilaterally cryptorchid adult rats, *Endocrinology,* 115, 550, 1984.

60. **Damber, J.-E., Bergh, A., Selstam, G., and Södergård, R.,** Estrogen receptor and aromatase activity in the testes of the unilateral cryptorchid rat, *Arch. Androl.,* 11, 259, 1983.

61. **Damber, J.-E. and Bergh, A.,** Decreased testicular response to acute LH-stimulation and increased intratesticular concentration of estradiol-17 beta in the abdominal testes in cryptorchid rats, *Acta Endocrinol.,* 95, 416, 1980.

62. **Rommerts, F. F. G., de Jong, F. H., Grootegoed, J. A., and van der Molen, H. J.,** Metabolic changes in testicular cells from rats after long-term exposure to 37°C in vivo or in vitro, *J. Endocrinol.,* 85, 471, 1980.

63. **Sharpe, R. M.,** Intratesticular factors controlling testicular function, *Biol. Reprod.,* 30, 29, 1984.

64. **Sharpe, R. M.,** Paracrine control of the testis, *Clin. Endocrinol. Metab.,* 15, 185, 1986.

65. **Saez, J. M., Tabone, E., Perrard-Sapori, M. H., and Rivarola, M. A.,** Paracrine role of Sertoli cells, *Med. Biol.,* 63, 225, 1985.

66. **Syed, V., Khan, S. A., and Ritzen, E. M.,** Stage-specific inhibition of interstitial cell testosterone secretion by rat seminiferous tubules in vitro, *Mol. Cell. Endocrinol.,* 40, 257, 1985.

67. **Bergh, A.,** Local differences in Leydig cell morphology in the adult rat testis — evidence for a local control of Leydig cells by adjacent seminiferous tubules, *Int. J. Androl.,* 5, 325, 1982.

68. **Bergh, A.,** Paracrine regulation of Leydig cells by the seminiferous tubules, *Int. J. Androl.,* 6, 57, 1983.

69. **Bergh, A. and Damber, J.-E.,** Local regulation of Leydig cells from the seminiferous tubules — effect of short-term cryptorchidism, *Int. J. Androl.,* 7, 409, 1984.

70. **Bergh, A. and Damber, J. E.,** HCG/LH-induced changes in testicular blood flow, microcirculation and vascular permeability in adult rats, in *Endocrinology and Physiology of Reproduction,* Armstrong, D. T., Friesch, H. G., Leung, P. C. K., Moger, W., and Ruf, K. B., Eds., Plenum Press, New York, in press.

71. **Bergh, A.,** Effect of cryptorchidism on the morphology of testicular macrophages — evidence for a Leydig cell macrophage interaction in the rat testis, *Int. J. Androl.,* 8, 86, 1985.

72. **Farrer, J. H., Sikka, S. C., Xie, H. W., Constantinide, D., and Rajfer, J.,** Impaired testosterone biosynthesis in cryptorchidism, *Fertil. Steril.,* 44, 125, 1985.

73. **Juenemann, K. P., Kogan, B. A., and Abozeid, M. H.,** Fertility in cryptorchidism: an experimental model, *J. Urol.,* 136, 214, 1986.

74. **Bergh, A. and Damber, J.-E.,** Morphological and endocrinological differences between abdominal testes in bilateral and unilateral cryptorchid rats, *Int. J. Androl.,* 2, 319, 1979.

75. **Jégou, B., Laws, A. O., and de Kretser, D. M.,** The effect of cryptorchidism and subsequent orchidopexy on testicular function in adult rats, *J. Reprod. Fertil.,* 69, 137, 1983.

76. **O'Leary, P., Jackson, A. E., Averill, S., and de Kretser, D. M.,** The effects of ethane dimethane sulphonate (EDS) on bilaterally cryptorchid rat testes, *Mol. Cell. Endocrinol.,* 45, 183, 1986.

77. **Karg, H. and Kronthaler, O.,** Histometrische untersuchungen am hormonproduzierenden Interstitialgewebe von Hoden kryptorchider tiere, *Zbl. Vet. Med.,* 7, 595, 1960.

78. **Straaten, H. W. M. and Wensing, C. J. G.,** Histomorphometric aspects of testicular morphogenesis in the naturally unilateral cryptorchid pig, *Biol. Reprod.,* 17, 473, 1977.

79. **Straaten, H. W. M., Ribbers-de Ridder, R., and Wensing, C. J. G.,** Early deviations of testicular Leydig cells in the naturally cryptorchid pig, *Biol. Reprod.,* 19, 171, 1978.

80. **Hadziselimovic, F.,** Cryptorchidism. Ultrastructure of normal and cryptorchid testis development, *Adv. Anat. Embryol. Cell Biol.,* 53, 3, 1977.

81. **Ezeasor, D. N.,** Light and electron microscopical observations on the Leydig cells of the scrotal and abdominal testes of naturally unilateral cryptorchid West African dwarf goats, *J. Anat.,* 141, 27, 1985.

82. **Sharpe, R. M., Doogan, D. G., and Cooper, I.,** Intratesticular factors and testosterone secretion: the role of luteinizing hormone in relation to changes during puberty and experimental cryptorchidism, *Endocrinology,* 119, 2089, 1986.

83. **Glover, T. D.,** Changes in blood flow in the testis and epididymis of the rat following artificial cryptorchidism, *Acta Endocrinol. (Kbh.),* Suppl. 100, 38, 1965.

84. **Hjertkvist, M., Bergh, A., and Damber, J. -E.,** HCG treatment increases intratesticular pressure in abdominal testes in unilaterally cryptorchid rats, *J. Androl.,* 9, 116, 1988.

85. **Bergh, A., Nikula, H., Damber, J.-E., Clayton, R., and Huhtaniemi, I.,** Altered concentrations of gonadotrophin, prolactin and GnRH receptors, and endogenous steroids in the abdominal testes of adult unilaterally cryptorchid rats, *J. Reprod. Fertil.,* 74, 279, 1985.

86. **de Kretser, D. M.,** Sertoli cell-Leydig cell interaction in regulation of testicular function, *Int. J. Androl.,* Suppl. 5, 11, 1982.

87. **Parvinen, M.,** Regulation of the seminiferous epithelium, *Endocr. Rev.,* 3, 404, 1982.

88. **Ritzén, E. M., Hansson, V., and French, F. S.,** The Sertoli cell, in *The Testis,* Burger, H. and de Kretser, D. M., Eds., Raven Press, New York, 1981, 171.

89. **Magueresse, B. L., Gac, F., Loir, M., and Jegou, B.,** Stimulation of rat Sertoli cell secretory activity in vitro by germ cells and residual bodies, *J. Reprod. Fertil.,* 77, 489, 1986.

90. **Galdieri, M. and Monaco, L. S.,** Secretion of androgen binding protein by Sertoli cells is influenced by contact with germ cells, *J. Androl.,* 5, 409, 1984.

91. **Vihko, K. K., Suominen, J. J. O., and Parvinen, M.,** Cellular regulation of plasminogen activator secretion during spermatogenesis, *Biol. Reprod.,* 31, 383, 1984.

92. **Chowdhury, A. K. and Steinberger, E.,** The influence of a cryptorchid milieu on the initiation of spermatogenesis in the rat, *J. Reprod. Fertil.,* 29, 173, 1972.

93. **Gomes, W. R. and Jain, S. K.,** Effect of unilateral and bilateral castration and cryptorchidism on serum gonadotrophins in the rat, *J. Endocrinol.,* 68, 191, 1976.

94. **Amatayakul, K., Ryan, R., Uozumi, T., and Albert, A.,** A reinvestigation of testicular-anterior pituitary relationships in the rat. I. Effects of castration and cryptorchidism, *Endocrinology,* 88, 872, 1971.

95. **Sharpe, R. M., Cooper, I., and Doogan, D. G.,** Increase in Leydig cell responsiveness in the unilaterally cryptorchid rat testis and its relationship to the intratesticular levels of testosterone, *J. Endocrinol.,* 102, 319, 1984.

96. **Jansz, G. F. and Pomerantz, D. K.,** A comparison of Leydig cell function after unilateral and bilateral cryptorchidism and efferent duct-ligation, *Biol. Reprod.,* 34, 316, 1986.

97. **Risbridger, G. P., Kerr, J. B., Peake, R., Rich, K. A., and de Kretser, D. M.,** Temporal changes in rat Leydig cell function after the induction of bilateral cryptorchidism, *J. Reprod. Fertil.,* 63, 415, 1981.

98. **Jahnsen, T., Gordeladze, J. O., Haug, E., and Hansson, V.,** Changes in rat testicular adenylate cyclase activities and gonadotrophin binding during unilateral experimental cryptorchidism, *J. Reprod. Fertil.,* 63, 381, 1981.

99. **Lloyd, B. J.,** Plasma testosterone and accessory sex glands in normal and cryptorchid rats, *J. Endocrinol.,* 54, 285, 1971.

100. **Antliff, H. R. and Young, W. C.,** Internal secretory capacity of the abdominal testis in the guinea pig, *Endocrinology,* 61, 121, 1957.

101. **Atkinson, P. M.,** The effects of early experimental cryptorchidism and subsequent orchidopexy on the maturation of the guinea-pig testicle, *Br. Surg.,* 60, 253, 1973.

102. **Skinner, J. D. and Rowson, L. E. A.,** Some effects of unilateral cryptorchism and vasectomy on sexual development of the pubescent ram and bull, *J. Endocrinol.,* 42, 311, 1968.

103. **Karpe, B., Hagenäs, L., Plöen, L., and Ritzéen, E. M.,** Studies on the scrotal testis in unilateral experimental cryptorchidism in rat and guinea pig, *J. Androl.,* 5, 59, 1982.

104. **Shirai, M., Matsushita, S., Kagayama, M., Ichijo, S., and Takeuchi, M.,** Histological changes of the scrotal testis in unilateral cryptorchidism, *Tohoku J. Exp. Med.,* 90, 363, 1966.

105. **Weifbach, I. B.,** Neue Aspekte zur Bedeutung und Behandlung von Hodendescensusstörungen, *Klin. Pädiat.,* 187, 289, 1975.

106. **Mengel, W., Moritz, P., Hüttmann, B., and Hecker, W. C.,** Investigations on pathogenesis of changes in descendes testes in unilateral cryptorchism, *Z. Kinderchir.,* 22, 369, 1977.

107. **Gottschalk, E., Friedrich, U., Meerbach, W., Müller, P., and Krech, K.,** Clinical and experimental studies of the problem of maldescended testis, *Z. Kinderchir.,* 22, 51, 1977.

108. **von Gärtner, K.,** Hereditärer kryptorchismus bei Wistarratten, *Z. Versuchstierk.,* 11, 179, 1969.

109. **Krause, H. H.,** Qualitative and quantitative investigations on spontaneously dystopic rat testicles, *Andrologie,* 4, 45, 1971.

110. **Nistal, M., Paniagua, R., and Queizan, A.,** Histologic lesions in undescended ectopic obstructed testes, *Fertil. Steril.,* 43, 455, 1985.

111. **Parvinen, M.,** Observations on freshly isolated and accurately identified spermatogenic cells of the rat. Early effects of heat and short-time experimental cryptorchidism, *Virchows Arch. B,* 13, 38, 1973.

112. **Plöen, L.,** An electron microscope study of the immediate effects on spermateleosis of a short-time experimental cryptorchidism in the rabbit, *Virchows Arch. B,* 10, 293, 1972.

113. **Plöen, L.,** An electron microscope study of the delayed effects on rabbit spermateleosis following experimental cryptorchidism for twenty-four hours, *Virchows Arch. B,* 14, 169, 1973.

114. **Plöen, L.,** A light microscope study of the immediate and delayed effects on rabbit spermatogenesis following experimental cryptorchidism for twenty-four hours, *Virchows Arch. B,* 14, 185, 1973.

115. **Lee, L. P. K. and Fritz, I. B.,** Studies on spermatogenesis in rats. V. Increased thermal lability of lysosomes from testicular germinal cells and its possible relationship to impairments in spermatogenesis in cryptorchidism, *J. Biol. Chem.,* 247, 7956, 1972.

116. **Nakamura, M., Romrell, L. J., and Hall, P. F.,** The effects of temperature and glucose on protein biosynthesis by immature (round) spermatids from rat testes, *J. Cell. Biol.,* 79, 1, 1978.

117. **Nakamura, M. and Hall, P. F.,** The mechanism by which body temperature inhibits protein biosynthesis in spermatids of rat testes, *J. Biol. Chem.,* 255, 2907, 1979.

118. **Hall, P. F., Kew, D., and Mita, M.,** The influence of temperature on the functions of cultured Sertoli cells, *Endocrinology,* 116, 1926, 1985.

119. **Knecht, H.,** Tubular structure and germ cell distribution of cryptorchid or normal testes in early childhood, *Beitr. Pathol.,* 159, 249, 1976.

120. **Gaudio, E., Paggiarino, D., and Carpino, F.,** Structural and ultrastructural modifications of cryptorchid human testes, *J. Urol.,* 131, 292, 1984.

121. **Straaten, H. W. M.,** Lack of a primary defect in maldescended testis of the neonatal pig, *Biol. Reprod.,* 19, 994, 1978.

122. **Fairfield, J.,** Effects of cold on infant rats; body temperature, oxygen consumption, electrocardiograms, *Am. J. Physiol.,* 155, 355, 1948.

123. **Battin, J. and Colle, M.,** Heterogeneite du syndrome "Cryptorchidie", *Arch. Franc. Ped.,* 34, 595, 1977.

124. **Scorer, C. G. and Farrington, G. H.,** *Congenital Deformities of the Testis and Epididymis,* Butterworth's, London, 1971.

125. **Hadziselimovic, F.,** Pathogenesis and treatment of undescended testes, *Eur. J. Pediatr.,* 139, 255, 1982.

126. **Raynaud, A.,** Inhibition sous l'effect d'unehormone oestogéne du development du gubernaculum du foetus male de souris, *C. R. Seance Acad. Sci. Paris,* 246, 176, 1958.

127. **Jean, C. L.,** Malformations génitales induites chez la souris adulte par une action oestogéne prénatale. I. Le male (pseudo-hermaphrodisme male), *Arch. Anat. Microsc. Morphol. Exp.,* 57, 121, 1968a.

128. **Habenicht, U. F. and Neumann, F.,** Hormonal regulation of testicular descent, *Adv. Anat. Embryol. Cell Biol.,* 81, 1981.

129. **Beard, C., Melton, L., O'Fallon, W., Noller, K. L., and Benson, R. C.,** Cryptorchism and maternal estrogen exposure, *Am. J. Epidemiol.,* 120, 707, 1984.

130. **Depue, R. H.,** Maternal gestational factors affecting the risk of cryptorchidism and inguinal hernia, *Int. J. Epidemiol.,* 13, 311, 1984.

131. **Pottern, L. M., Brown, L. M., Hoover, R. N., Javadpour, N., O'Conell, W. J., Stutzman, R. E., and Blattner, W. A.,** Testicular cancer risk among young men: role of cryptorchidism and inguinal hernia, *J. Natl. Cancer Inst.,* 74, 377, 1985.

132. **Davies, T. W., Williams, D. R. R., and Whitaker, R. H.,** Risk factors for undescended testis, *Int. J. Epidemiol.,* 15, 197, 1986.

133. **McEwen, B. S.,** Gonadal steroids and brain development, *Biol. Reprod.,* 22, 43, 1980.

134. **Gaytan, F., Pinilla, L., Aguilar, R., Lucena, M. C., and Paniagua, R.,** Effects of neonatal estrogen administration on rat testis development with particular reference to Sertoli cells, *J. Androl.,* 7, 112, 1986.

135. **Bellido, C., Gaytan, A. R., Pinilla, L., and Aguilar, E.,** Prepuberal reproductive defects in neonatal estrogenized male rats, *Biol. Reprod.,* 53, 381, 1985.

136. **Jean, C. L.,** Malformations génitales induites chez la souris adulte par une action oestrogéne prenatale. II. La femelle, *Arch. Anat. Microsc. Morphol. Exp.,* 57, 191, 1968b.

137. **Nishimune, Y., Aizawa, S., and Komatsu, T.,** Testicular germ cell differentiation in vivo, *Fertil. Steril.,* 29, 95, 1978.

138. **Kormano, M., Härkönen, M., and Kontinen, E.,** Effect of experimental cryptorchidism on the histochemically demonstrable dehydrogenases of the rat testis, *Endocrinology,* 74, 44, 1964.

139. **Davis, J. T. and Coniglio, J. G.,** The effect of cryptorchidism, cadmium and anti-spermatogenic drugs on fatty acid composition of rat testis, *J. Reprod. Fertil.,* 14, 407, 1967.

140. **Keel, B. A. and Abney, T. O.,** Alterations of testicular function in the unilaterally cryptorchid rat, *Proc. Exp. Soc. Biol. Med.,* 166, 489, 1981.

141. **Aumüller, G., Hartmann, K., Giers, U., and Schenck, B.,** Fine structure of the Sertoli cells of the rat testis in experimental unilateral cryptorchidism, *Int. J. Androl.,* 3, 301, 1980.

Chapter 3

ALTERATIONS IN THE STEROIDOGENIC CAPACITY OF LEYDIG CELLS IN CRYPTORCHID TESTIS

Friedrich Jockenhovel and Ronald S. Swerdloff

TABLE OF CONTENTS

I. INTRODUCTION

Cryptorchidism is a well-known cause of impaired spermatogenesis. Bilateral cryptorchidism, when uncorrected until adulthood, is a predictive cause of male factor infertility. It is now recognized that the temperature-dependent effects of nondescent of the testis can produce damage to the germinal elements considerably before sexual maturation is complete. In addition, there are data which suggest that some patients with cryptorchidism have predisposing abnormalities in the reproductive hormone axis including hypogonadotropic hypogonadism and primary testicular damage. In contrast to the obvious effects of cryptorchidism on the germinal tubules, its effects on testicular steroidogenesis remain controversial. This chapter will present the evidence on this topic in the framework of the normal steroidogenic developmental process.

Normal testicular descent is characterized by the migration of the testis and epididymis from an abdominal position into the scrotum (see Chapter 1). This process normally occurs within the last trimester of gestation. Within the first 7 months of gestation, the testis migrates to a position just above the internal inguinal ring. In the remaining months of intrauterine life, the testis descends through the inguinal canal into the scrotum. Several hypotheses have been postulated in an attempt to explain the mechanical factors leading to testicular descent, among which the abdominal pressure, epididymal push, and hormonal factor theories are most favored. Engle and Hamilton[1,2] showed more than 50 years ago, that pregnancy serum and testosterone both can mediate testicular descent. In subsequent studies, Rajfer and Walsh demonstrated that high local concentrations of dihydrotestosterone are required to promote testicular descent.[3] Based on these and other studies, a model of hormonal regulation of testicular descent has been proposed. The hypothalamus secretes gonadotropin releasing hormone (GnRH) which stimulates the pituitary to synthesize and release follicle stimulating hormone (FSH) and luteinizing hormone (LH). The gonadotropins, in turn, stimulate the Leydig cell to produce testosterone, which is converted to dihydrotestosterone by 5-alpha reductase within the testis and in the target tissue. At this point, the assumption is made that androgens and, in particular, dihydrotestosterone somehow influence the gubernaculum testis, the epididymis or other structures involved in testicular descent to facilitate the migration of the testis through the inguinal canal into the scrotum. This hypothesis is strongly supported by clinical observations. A large variety of disorders which interfere with the hypothalamus-pituitary-testicular axis can cause cryptorchidism. To give a few examples, anencephaly, Kallman's syndrome, pituitary aplasia, and the testicular enzyme deficiencies, (3-beta-hydroxysteroid dehydrogenase and 17,20-desmolase deficiency) are all able to cause cryptorchidism.

However, another clinical observation casts doubt on the hypothesis that testicular descent is regulated purely by androgens. Testicular feminization syndrome is caused by the absence of androgen receptors in target tissues. According to the current model, patients bearing this syndrome should have cryptorchid testis. In reality, the majority of the patients have descended testis, either in the labira majora or at least in the inguinal canal.[4,5] In experimental cryptorchidism, antiandrogens interfere with testicular descent, but do not completely inhibit it.[6,7] These observations have led to the hypothesis that additional hormonal factors play an important role in the testicular descent. There are indications that Müllerian inhibiting substance (MIS) is responsible for the intraabdominal migration, but this needs further confirmation.[8-10]

In addition to the aforementioned diseases causing cryptorchidism, a great variety of genetic and anatomical disturbances are associated with maldescent of the testes. However, in 80 to 90% of all cases the pathogenic basis for cryptorchidism is not revealed. In these patients with isolated cryptorchidism, all organs involved in the development of male reproductive function can possibly be responsible for the undescended testis. Therefore, isolated cryptorchidism most likely represents a variety of disturbances, all capable of causing the same symptoms. Furthermore, studying cryptorchid patients postnatally may not be helpful in identifying possible differences to a normal population, since any alterations might be transient and limited to a short time period during intrauterine life. As long as we do not have the diagnostic criteria to discriminate between varieties of isolated cryptorchidism, boys with this disease represent a very heterogeneous study population. Data obtained from this mixed group will not give a definitive answer.

II. STEROIDOGENESIS IN INFANCY

Forest et al.[11] were the first to discover testicular activity during the first year of life of normal infants. At birth, the testosterone levels in cord blood are between 0.2 and 0.36 μg/ ml[11-14] and about tenfold higher in the peripheral circulation.[13,15,16] At this time there are no differences between normal and cryptorchid newborns. In the normal male infant a rapid decrease in plasma levels of dehydroepiandrosterone, testosterone, and dihydrotestosterone occurs within the first 2 weeks of life. This decline is the result of the declining levels of maternal human chorionic gonadotropin (hCG) becoming undetectable 5 d after birth.[17] These lowered testosterone levels are followed by a gradual increase during the 2nd and 3rd months of life to 2 to 3 ng/ml, levels equal to early and mid-puberty.[11,13,14,18,19] This increase in testosterone is associated with a rise in plasma luteinizing hormone (LH),[11,18,20] suggesting that increased secretion of LH by the pituitary leads to stimulation of testosterone production by the testis. The metabolic clearance rate of androgens has not been studied in infants, therefore changes in testosterone degradation could theoretically be a factor in the increased blood levels. Agonadal boys do not demonstrate the rise in testosterone between days 30 and 90, proving a gonadal source of the testosterone at this time.[21] Pregnenolone, dehydroepiandrosterone, and 5-alpha-dihydrotestosterone are also elevated during this period.[16,22] Therefore, it seems that neonatal testicular steroidogenesis occurs via the delta-5-pathway, as it does in adult men,[23,25] (Figure 1) and that peripheral conversion of testosterone to 5-alpha-dihydrotestosterone occurs in infants. On the other hand, 17-alpha-hydroxyprogesterone, androstenedione, and androsterone are also elevated, but since there are only minor differences between male and female serum concentrations with no correlation between age and androstenedione, they are more likely to be secreted by the adrenals.[16,22] The physiologic meaning, if any, of this androgen surge in early infancy has not been elucidated. After the 3rd month, androgen levels decline, reaching prepubertal values between the 7th and 12th months after birth,[11] accompanied by decreased basal and GnRH mobilizable LH levels.[20]

In both uni- or bilateral cryptorchid boys, the testosterone plasma levels exhibit the same pattern, but with a significant attenuation of the surge between days 30 and 90. Testosterone concentrations reach only 50% of the levels of normal boys.[26,27] It is interesting to note that cryptorchid infants in whom spontaneous migration of one or both testes into the scrotum occurred within 4 months after birth, testosterone levels were similar to normal children, suggesting either heterogeneity in the disease[26] or the likelihood that retractile testes are a variant of normal (Figure 2).[28] The study by Gendrel et al.[26] did not clarify whether a deficiency in the response of the Leydig cell to adequate stimulation by LH or a lack of LH secretion caused the lower testosterone levels in cryptorchid babies, since LH was not measured. A diminished LH secretion was considered to be more likely since the release of LH by the pituitary is significantly reduced in cryptorchid infants, as revealed by GnRH stimulation tests.[29,30] The reports on basal LH levels are contradictory though, some finding lower LH values in cryptorchid boys;[29,31] others finding no significant differences.[27,32] The discrepancies could be due to a different number of patients in the critical age of 2 to 3 months or heterogeneity in the various study populations. The hypothesis that reduced stimulation by LH rather than impaired response of the Leydig cell leads to the attenuated

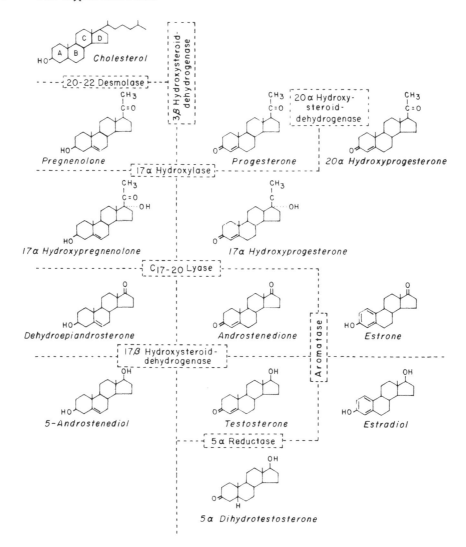

FIGURE 1.   Comparison of testosterone serum levels (ng/ml) in boys 12- to 180- d of age with bilateral and unilateral cryptorchidism to levels in boys with postnatal spontaneous migration into the scrotum (bilateral, unilateral) and to a normal range (shaded area). For true cryptorchid boys and boys with delayed spontaneous migration (---) a polynomial regression curve is given (From Gendrel, D., Job, J.-C., and Roger, M., *Acta Endocrinol.*, 89, 372, 1978. With permission.)

testosterone rise is further nourished by the observation that there are no differences between uni- or bilateral cryptorchid infants regarding their testosterone levels.[26] It has not been evaluated whether LH is secreted in a pulsatile fashion at this age, as is well established in puberty and adulthood,[33] and neither of these studies has used pooled serum samples or measured LH in several samples drawn 10 to 20 min apart from each other. The possibility that the LH and testosterone peaks might have been missed cannot be ruled out.

Leydig cell stimulation tests in cryptorchid infants within the 1st year of life showed a tenfold increase in testosterone secretion, after intramuscular injection of 500 I.U. hCG every other day for 6 d, as compared to basal levels.[29,32] For ethical reasons, healthy infants of this age group were not available as controls. Studies in healthy, prepubertal children, older than 1 year, also showed a tenfold increase of testosterone levels after hCG stimulation, thus suggesting that these data in cryptorchid children less than 1 year may be a normal response.[34-38]

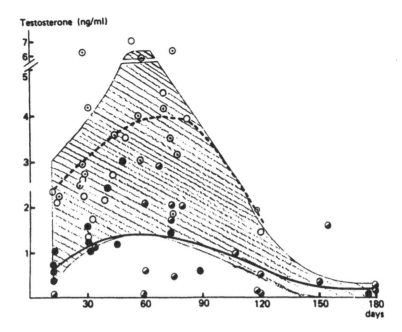

FIGURE 2. Comparison of testosterone serum levels (ng/ml) in boys 12- to 180-d of age with bilateral (●) and unilateral (◑) cryptorchidism to levels in boys with postnatal spontaneous migration into the scrotum (bilateral [⊙], unilateral [○] and to a normal range (shaded area). ——— is the polynomial regression curve in cryptorchids. ----- is the polynomial regression curve in boys with delayed spontaneous testicular descent. (From Gendrel, D., Job, J.-C., and Roger, M., *Acta Endocrinol.*, 89, 372, 1978. With permission.)

The significant increase of testosterone secretion after hCG stimulation coupled with a diminished LH response to GnRH stimulation test implies, at least partly, an insufficiency of either the pituitary or higher structures, such as the hypothalamus. However, this hypogonadotrophic hypogonadism has to be functional and transient, since the majority of cryptorchid adults lack such a disorder.

In contrast to this hypothesis, Facchinetti et al.[27] reported evidence for direct impairment of Leydig cell function in cryptorchid infants. These investigators found normal basal LH levels in cryptorchid babies during the critical age period of 2 to 3 months and confirmed the data by Gendrel et al.[26] regarding the attenuated testosterone levels. At the same time, dehydroepiandrosterone levels were in a similar range as that of healthy infants, suggesting decreased activity of the enzymes delta-5-3-beta and 17-beta-hydroxysteroid dehydrogenase, both responsible for conversion of dehydroepiandrosterone to testosterone (Figure 1). However, the number of individuals studied by Facchinetti et al.[27] is too small to draw a final conclusion. Their findings are substantiated by data obtained in rats. In experimental cryptorchidism, the delta-5-3-beta hydroxysteroid dehydrogenase is known to be heat-sensitive when exposed to higher temperatures for a prolonged period of time.[40-43] Data on the temperature sensitivity of the 17-beta hydroxydehydrogenase are still controversial.[40,44,45] In rat testicular steroidogenesis, the major pathway is the delta-4 pathway, via progesterone, 17-alpha-hydroxyprogesterone and androstenedione,[46] and one has to be very cautious in extrapolating data gained in rats to men.

Morphological studies did not resolve the question of the cause of the lowered testosterone levels in cryptorchid infants. In contrast to Hayashi and Harrison,[40] who applied light microscopy, Hadziselimovic,[48] using an electron microscope, was able to identify Leydig cells in the interstitium of infants with cryptorchid testis. The Leydig cells were hypo- or atrophic showing irregular shaped nuclei, fewer mitochondria and very scarce smooth endoplasmic reticulum, compared to controls of the same age, indicating a diminished functional activity. Some Leydig cells even underwent degeneration.[49] In healthy infants of this age group, the Leydig cell is well developed and rich in endoplasmic reticulum.[50,51] The number of Leydig cells, expressed per tubule, is significantly higher throughout the first 5 months of life in normal testis, compared to biopsies from cryptorchid children.[52]

Therefore, carefully designed and detailed future studies are necessary to clarify the cause of the attenuated transient testosterone rise in cryptorchid boys in the 1st year of life. One might speculate that altered LH secretion influences the activity of enzymes in the steroidogenic pathway. For example, constant instead of pulsatile LH release would thereby explain the reduced releasable LH stores of the pituitary. In rat *in vivo* and *in vitro* experiments,[53-58] as well as in men,[59-62] it is well established that steroidogenic response to hCG is not only dose dependent, but is influenced by the mode of application. Constant low doses of LH can lead to Leydig cell desensitization, leading to reduced enzyme activity and decreased steroidogenesis.

All studies assessing LH activities in the serum of cryptorchid neonates and infants measured only the immunoactivity rather than bioactivity of LH. From studies interfering with the hypothalamic-pituitary axis by means of application of GnRH analogs, it is known that the ratio between bioactivity and immunoactivity of LH can be greatly reduced.[63-65] At this time it cannot be excluded that at least a subgroup of cryptorchid patients has a lowered LH bioactivity in the presence of normal or only moderately lowered immunoactive LH. On the other hand, it is difficult to favor the hypothesis of LH insufficiency in view of the lack of hypogonadotrophic hypogonadism in cryptorchid adults. In the presence of strong evidence for decreased enzyme activity of the steroidogenic pathway in experimental cryptorchidism and an indication that this is also true in human subjects, it seems very likely that decreased testosterone levels are a reflection of impaired Leydig cell function.

III. STEROIDOGENESIS IN CHILDHOOD

During childhood, testicular steroidogenesis is at rest and secretion of testosterone and other androgens is very low and shows no sex differences.[19] The levels of plasma testosterone in normal prepubertal boys younger than 6 years is around 0.05 ng/ml.[13,66-68] Most of these androgens seem to be from adrenal sources,[68,69] but the testis is actively secreting steroids, as is evidenced by gradients between cubital vein and spermatic vein plasma levels of progesterone, 17-alpha-hydroxyprogesterone and 20-alpha-dihydroprogesterone.[70]

It is widely accepted that basal testosterone levels are similar in healthy boys and in boys with one or two undescended testes,[29,35,37,39,69,71-82] though there are reports finding higher[83] or lower levels.[74] One report, finding lower levels in cryptorchid testis, is inconclusive as the authors find normal amounts of testosterone in urine despite lower blood levels.[64] Only two of these studies observed significant differences between uni- and bilateral cryptorchid boys, finding 0.38 ± 0.09 ng/ml and 0.79 ± 0.10 ng/ml in unilateral and 0.22 ± 0.12 ng/ml and 0.29 ± 0.05 ng/ml in bilateral cryptorchid children.[75,81] All values can be considered to be in the normal range for healthy prepubertal boys,[66,67] and only a few subjects were studied (eight bilateral cryptorchid boys in both studies).

Furthermore, since there are no indications of altered testosterone secretion in prepubertal cryptorchid children and no clinical signs of androgen deficiency, the differences which might exist seem not to be physiologically significant. Whereas information on plasma levels of testosterone is abundant, other steroids have, in general, not been measured. Only very few studies have assessed the levels of testosterone precursors or metabolites. Steroids of the delta-4-pathway, i.e., 17-alpha-hydroxyprogesterone and androstenedione[64,73,75] as well as steroids of the delta-5-pathway (dihydroepiandrosterone and dihydroepiandrosterone sulfate)[75,79] are in the normal range (Figure 1). At this age, circulating dihydroepiandrosterone and its sulfate are more likely to originate from the adrenals. The activity of the 5-alpha-reductase in the gonads and other peripheral sites is not altered as evidenced by normal levels of dihydrotestosterone.[79] Information on 17-beta-estradiol is inconclusive. Two studies report normal values,[81,82] one indicates higher levels in cryptorchid children (30.5 ± 24.9 vs. 21.1 ± 6.8 pg/ml), but was not able to prove a significant difference because of the high standard deviation in the cryptorchid group.[76] Some of the cryptorchid children demonstrated elevated levels of 17-beta-estradiol. This study included boys of an advanced age (13 years); therefore, onset of puberty could have interfered with increased estradiol levels reflecting hyperstimulation of the testis by elevated levels of serum LH.[80]

Numerous studies have evaluated the Leydig cell function in response to stimulation tests (see Table 1). The results are not uniform. The response of the Leydig cell to hCG stimulation, as evaluated by comparison of basal vs. stimulated values was found to be higher,[39] normal,[37,84] or lower[36,69,79,80] in cryptorchid testis (see Table 1). Different protocols, different doses of hCG over different time periods, and different ages of the patients make comparisons difficult. All studies excluded patients with previous hCG therapy. Some authors consider uni- or bilateral cryptorchid children as one group, not observing differences between them,[29,32,37,85-87] while others find a lower response to hCG stimulation only in bilateral cryptorchidism.[34,35,72,75] Forest et al.[88] showed that timing of blood sampling after the last hCG injection is crucial as the maximal testosterone response to hCG was measured 72 to 120 h after either one or two hCG injections, preceded by a smaller peak 4 to 6 h after the injections. Most studies collected blood 24 h after the last injection of hCG,[29,32,34,36,39,69,73,75,79,80,85,89] others 72 h[90] or 96 h[37] later. One study does not mention time of blood drawing.[72] In interpretation of the data, it is also important to be aware of the age of the patients.

The onset of puberty, assessed by clinical signs as defined by Marshall and Tanner,[91] is preceded by a gradual increase of androgens which leads to the morphological changes occurring in puberty. As early as 6 years of age, slowly rising androgen levels can be observed,[92] which are secreted by the adrenals, as evidenced by dexamethasone suppression and ACTH stimulation.[89] The pubertal increase in testicular testosterone secretion in general does not begin until the age of ten.[68,88] The gradual rise in the response to gonadotropin stimulation, observed in the rat,[94] has also been demonstrated to occur in the child.[34,39,77,78,84,87,89] Therefore, a broad age range can lead to misinterpretation of the data.

The most critical points are the dosage and the timing of injection. The hCG dose ranges from 800 to 5000 I.U. per single injection and from 1000 to 12,000 I.U. in cumulative doses. Very high doses or extensive periods of stimulation extinguish differences between cryptorchid and normal children.[87] The time period over which the stimulation was performed stretches from 1 d to 6 weeks and seems to be even more important than the cumulative dose.[72] These different regimens make comparisons very difficult, if not impossible, and can certainly account for the above-mentioned discrepancies. Only two studies adjust the hCG dose to the body size.[37,73] All other studies applied the same dose of hCG to all children, thereby inevitably over- or underdosing some of the patients. Obviously, too-low doses cannot give a maximal response. Overdosing, however, can lead to Leydig cell refractoriness, leaving the Leydig cell unable to respond adequately.[88]

From the vast amount of data gathered, one can draw the conclusion that in many children with undescended testes the response of the Leydig cell to hCG is diminished, compared to normal children. But there are also cryptorchid boys showing a normal response, with a higher incidence among unilateral cryptorchidism.[35,36,39,69] This reflects the heterogeneity of cryptorchid children, as well as the different protocols and regimens. Leitz et al.[95] clearly demonstrated that almost two thirds of his cryptorchid study group had a normal (two standard deviations above or below the mean of 5.54 ± 1.21 ng/ml in healthy prepubertal boys) response to hCG. Grant et al.[36] obtained similar results in 50% of his patients. Most authors

Table 1

SERUM TESTOSTERONE LEVELS IN PREPUBERTAL CRYPTORCHID BOYS BEFORE AND AFTER hCG STIMULATION

hCG Dose (IU) and Regimen	Groups	Plasma T in ng/dl		Age (range)	n	Ref.
		Basal	Stimulated			
2000 single dose	Control	18 ± 4	61 ± 16	5.5—9	8	39
	Bi	50 ± 30	184 ± 46	4—16	4	39
2000 daily for	Control	18 ± 4	173 ± 27	5.5—9	8	39
3 d	Bi	50 ± 30	255 ± 58	4—16	4	39
5000/1.7 m² single dose	Uni + bi	3 ± 1	213 ± 57	1.7—10.4	8	73
800—5000 daily for	Uni	26 ± 24	431 ± 96	4—11	13	72
5 d	Bi	43 ± 28	329 ± 172	4—11	16	72
1500 every 2 d	Control	14 ± 2	337 ± 43	x = 8.5 ± 0.4	24	83
for 6 d	Uni + bi	15 ± 13	140 ± 111		11	83
1500 every 2 d	Control	16 ± 3	1061 ± 711	Puberty	4	83
for 18 d	Uni + bi	15 ± 13	724 ± 451	Stage P_1	11	83
1500 every 2 d for 6 d	Uni + bi	12 ± 1	210 ± 12	1—13	107	29
1500 every 2 d	Uni	31 ± 36	266 ± 61	4—13.5	26	
for 6 d	Bi	16 ± 4	154 ± 32			85
1500 daily for 3 d	Control	14 ± 16	337 ± 43	Puberty	24	86
	Bi + uni	0.13 ± 1	185 ± 132	Stage P_1	79	86
2000 daily for 3 d[a]	Normal	30 ± 16	139 ± 28	7.3—12	26	98
	Uni + bi	29 ± 10	99 ± 41	6.8—11.8	8	98
1500 daily for 3 d	Control	15 ± 6	166 ± 36	12.2—10.7	18	34
	Uni	17 ± 6	173 ± 43	3.1—11	18	34
	Bi	14 ± 8	131 ± 49	3.3—11.5	17	34
1500 daily for 3 d	Control	145 ± 106	488 ± 270	7—13	43	80
	Bi + uni	87 ± 77	349 ± 210	8—13	51	80
5000/m² single dose	Uni	82 ± 17	278 ± 52[b]	7.1 ± 12.6	12	90
	Bi	99 ± 20	302 ± 37	4.7 ± 12.6	10	90
2000 daily for 3 days	Control	15 ± 1[c]	114 ± 10[c]	4.8—11.7	22	35
	Uni	20 ± 2	91 ± 8	4.8—11.2	33	35
	Bi	15 ± 2	78 ± 12	4.0—11.3	14	35
2 × 5000/1.7 m² 4 d apart	Uni + bi	7.2[d]	418	0.6—6.1	9	84
5000/1.7 m²[e]	Uni + bi	5.8[d]	498[f]	1.1—12.4	16	84
1500 daily for 5 d	Control	45 ± 9	360 ± 50	5—12	8	79
	Uni	46 ± 5	261 ± 78	3—12	11	79
2000 daily for 4 d	Uni	71 ± 10	315 ± 28	1.6—13.0	24	16
	Bi	29 ± 5	206 ± 37	1.6—13.0	8	16
3000 daily for 3 d	Uni	38 ± 9	123 ± 31	6.5—11.7	10	81
	Bi	22 ± 12	147 ± 44	6.5—11.7	8	81
10,000/m² body surface single	Control	25 ± 10[d]	250 ± 50[d]	7.6—9.3	10	37
dose	Uni	25 ± 10	270 ± 50	7.0—9.6	18	37
	Bi	25 ± 10	225 ± 50[f]	7.3—9.6	17	37
1500 every 2 d for 14 d	Control	32 ± 10	554 ± 121	2—13.4	16	38
1500 every 2 d for 14 d	Control	7 ± 3	614 ± 240	1—8	45	69
	Uni + bi	Normal	474 ± 450	1—13.6	106	69
1000 twice a week for 6	Bi	28 ± 17	267 ± 104	5—11	27	77
weeks	Uni	26 ± 11	253 ± 72	5—11	11	77

Note: Bi = bilateral cryptorchidism; Uni = unilateral cryptorchidism; Un: + bi = both bilateral and unilateral cryptorchidism.

[a]   Previous treatment with 20 mg dexamethasone/d for 6 d and in addition to hCG.
[b]   Samples drawn 3 d after injection.
[c] $x \pm$ SEM.
[d]   Estimated from figure.
[e]   Injections on days 0, 4, 7, and 10.
[f]   Samples drawn 4 d after injection.

agree that there is considerable variation in the response to stimulation. The higher incidence of normal response in unilateral cryptorchidism can be explained by a compensation of lower secretion of the undescended testis by the contralateral descended testis.[91,92]

The response of other steroids to hCG stimulation has only rarely been measured. Androgens like androstenedione or dehydroepiandrosterone show a much lesser increase than testosterone,[75] whereas 5-alpha-dihydrotestosterone exhibits a significant and prolonged rise.[73,97] Tapanainen et al.[73] observed a sharp increase of 5-alpha-dihydrotestosterone 48 h after a single injection of 5000 I.U. hCG/1.7 m^2 body surface, with a peak threefold higher than basal levels after 120 h. A treatment of two injections per week of 1000 I.U. hCG each, for 6 weeks, also resulted in a threefold increase at the end of the treatment period.[97] The difference in the basal and peak levels between these studies can be explained by assay differences and the fact that Attanasio et al.[97] studied an older age group than Tapanainen et al.[73] (5.9 ± 2.85 years vs. 8.43 ± 1.9 years, respectively).

Estradiol shows a biphasic pattern. After an initial decrease 6 h after the first injection of hCG,[73] 17-beta-estradiol returns to the baseline at 24 h[80,86,87,89,90] and then shows a gradual but steady increase after a third injection of hCG on day 7[84]. This is an agreement with Toublanc et al.[89] who demonstrated that estrogens increase slowly during the process of puberty as a result of Leydig cell maturation. There are no significant differences between cryptorchid or healthy boys in regard to estrogen levels, but few individuals with undescended testes have higher estradiol levels.[80,89]

The progestin, 17-β-hydroxyprogesterone, exhibits a similar pattern to 17-beta-estradiol, also showing an initial decrease and then a slow increase which continued for 2 weeks after the first of four hCG injections (the last injection was given on day 10).[73,84] Other gestagens, like pregnenolone and progesterone, demonstrated a 50% reduction 36 h after a single hCG injection. Data on healthy boys are not available, therefore it is not possible to make any comparisons. But there are no obvious defects.

In vitro studies with human testicular tissue of undescended testis did not show any significant differences to normal prepubertal boys. The metabolism of radioactive-labeled progesterone and its conversion into other steroids did not differ significantly in normal or cryptorchid tissue,[99-101] though there seems to be the tendency toward a quantitative lower conversion to 17-alpha-hydroxyprogesterone in tissue from cryptorchid testis. This conversion is not significant due to a large variation of the amount produced by the normal tissue.[99,100] The LH receptor function has been assessed by incubation of biopsy specimen with LH and the subsequent measurement of cAMP production, which did not reveal any differences between the undescended and the descended testis.[102] However, an underlying defect in both testes cannot be ruled out. Lackgren et al.[103] found specific, but low binding of LH in prepubertal cryptorchid testes. Since normal boys were not studied, no statement on alteration is possible. In contrast, in the surgically cryptorchid rat changes in the binding capacity for LH occur. The total number of LH as well as of FSH and prolactin receptors, expressed per testis or per Leydig cell, is reduced by 40 to 70%.[56,104-109] Whether this is true for the human remains to be established. It is well known that the number of LH receptors per Leydig cell by far exceeds the number needed for maximal stimulation.[110,111] Therefore, a reduction of the membrane receptors for LH might not play a decisive role in the diminished testosterone response to hCG stimulation.

Morphological studies do not give much additional information since Leydig cells are rarely seen in the interstitium between infancy and puberty. The few Leydig cells visible in healthy boys are smaller than Leydig cells in infancy. The nucleus is well developed and the smooth endoplasmic reticulum fills almost the entire cell. Only a few lipoid droplets can be observed.[112] In the cryptorchid testis the nucleus is irregular, the lipoid droplets are more frequent and the smooth endoplasmic reticulum is scarce.[51,113] In contrast, the rough endoplasmic reticulum is well developed.[113] This is in agreement with Sohval,[50] who did not recognize well-differentiated Leydig cells in cryptorchid testis of this age group either.

Numanoglu et al.[114] observed a progressive degeneration of Leydig cells in cryptorchid testis after the age of 5 years.

In conclusion, except for a blunted testosterone response to hCG, there is no evidence for altered steroidogenesis in the cryptorchid testis prior to puberty. But does this diminished response to a stimulation test have any significant meaning? Prepubertal and pubertal development proceeds normally in cryptorchid boys and does not reveal any sign of androgen deficiency. On the other hand, the role of androgens in initiation of spermatogenesis is well accepted, and it is also well known that spermatogenesis is greatly reduced in most cryptorchid patients, as will be pointed out elsewhere in this book (Chapter 9). It is not clear whether a local androgen deficiency in the testis can account at least in part, for the reduced spermatogenesis.

The cause for the lower testosterone response to hCG stimulation seems to be at a higher level, as was shown by Gendrel et al.[29] Pretreatment of cryptorchid boys with hCG, which did not result in descent of the testis, cancelled out the difference in response to a stimulation test as compared to normal boys. hCG therapy also leads to increased LH binding in undescended testis[103] and increased the amount of 17-alpha-hydroxyprogesterone produced from progesterone in *in vitro* studies, as well as the amount of endoplasmic reticulum and the number of mitochondria.[48,116] This suggests that a defect at the level of the pituitary or the hypothalamus, leading to lower stimulation of the Leydig cells by gonadotropins is responsible for the diminished capacity of the Leydig cells. This is an agreement with findings in LHRH tests, demonstrating a lower LH response in many studies[29,78,80,81,117] and the good correlation between peak LH and peak testosterone values in stimulation tests.[28,112]

IV. STEROIDOGENESIS IN PUBERTY

An introduction into the development of puberty in normal male children is well beyond the scope of this chapter. Reviews on this subject include those of Swerdloff and Heber[33] and Forest et al.[21] In brief, puberty begins with gradually increasing gonadotropin levels. This increase is most likely due to changes at the hypothalamic-pituitary axis. These changes may reflect decreased inhibitory neurotransmitter input at the hypothalamus or decreased sensitivity on the gonadostat in the hypothalamus to the negative feedback by steroids, leading to increased GnRH output. At the same time the pituitary response to GnRH increases. Both factors contribute to a steady rise of the gonadotropin levels, which in the beginning are secreted in large nocturnal pulses.[119,120] As puberty advances these pulses occur during the day, too. The higher levels of LH stimulate the Leydig cell to increase androgen production. This process is supported by the rising responsiveness of the testis to gonadotrophic stimulation.[21,33,94] The elevated androgen levels lead to the clinical changes occurring during puberty.

Studies on the endocrine function of undescended testis in adolescence are not as frequent as in childhood, and usually involve a smaller number of individuals, since most children of this age have, fortunately, undergone orchidopexy. As pointed out earlier, puberty proceeds normally in cryptorchid children as assessed by clinical signs of puberty (pubic hair distribution, penile length and somatic growth),[121] though there are indications that at least in a subgroup of cryptorchid patients the somatic growth might be slightly altered.[122] A careful examination by Canlorbe et al.[86] and Gendrel et al.[29] revealed that in the early stage of puberty (P_2 according to Marshall and Tanner[91]), the response of the Leydig cell to hCG stimulation is blunted, as it is in childhood. In mid-puberty this response becomes normal.[29,86] Basal values of testosterone are in the normal range in one study,[29] but are retarded in early pubertal stages in another and become normal at late puberty.[86] Estrogens exhibited the same pattern: normal basal values, diminished peak concentration after hCG in puberty stage P_2 which becomes normal in all later stages.[82] A retardation of the pubertal increase in urinary testosterone excretion was also observed.[83] Other studies could not confirm these results, because they group the subjects by chronological age instead of puberty stages,[74] include different puberty stages in one group,[37] study a small number of individuals,[73] or include undescended testes with other testicular abnormalities in the same group.[84,90] As Gendrel et al.[29] obtained parallel results in GnRH stimulation tests and in the hCG test, i.e., a blunted response of LH in early puberty, which becomes normal in mid-puberty, they suggest a defect at the hypothalamic or pituitary level. This leads to insufficient Leydig cell stimulation, leaving the testis unable to produce adequate responses in hCG stimulation tests. This is consistent with the observation made during cryptorchidism in childhood. The defect seems to be overcome at mid-puberty. These results have been confirmed in part by Dickermann et al.[120] They also observed a decreased response to hCG stimulation in early puberty, but could not demonstrate a normal response at mid- or end puberty. This discrepancy can be explained by the different hCG doses used and the time lapse between injection of hCG and the blood drawings. Whereas Gendrel et al.[29] and Canlorbe et al.[86] injected 3 × 1500 I.U. hCG every second day for 5 d and drew blood on day 6, Dickermann et al.[121] gave a single dose of 5000 I.U. hCG and took blood 96 h after the injection.

The retarded maturation of the hypothalamic-pituitary-testicular axis in the cryptorchid testis, as proposed by Gendrel et al.[29] and Canlorbe et al.,[86] finds its reflection in histological investigations. In light and electron microscopy, a clearly delayed maturation of the Leydig cell is evident.[48,112,114,123] This finding is not only in regard to the cell number, but also to reduced smooth and rough endoplasmic reticulum, scarce mitochondria, and poorly developed Golgi apparatus.[124] Hayashi and Harrison[47] observed the reappearance of Leydig cells in normal boys in the 5th year, whereas in undescended testes, Leydig cells were completely absent until the 10th year of age. Some Leydig cells undergo progressive degeneration.

However, there are authors who did not see these alterations in cryptorchid testes and state that the pubertal differentiation of Leydig cells in the undescended testis proceeds normally, with a large variation in individual numbers of Leydig cells.[50,125] Their findings substantiate observations made in *in vitro* studies. Pasqualini et al.[126] found adult levels of intratesticular testosterone during early puberty in biopsies of cryptorchid testes, with an increased ratio between intratesticular and serum testosterone, suggesting that the testosterone is not secreted into the circulation. However, the wide range of intratesticular testosterone levels in the six pubertal cryptorchid boys studied (37 to 1352 ng/g tissue), with at least one patient clearly having prepubertal levels, may reflect the heterogeneity of cryptorchidism or a case of delayed onset of puberty. The other five patients obviously have adult levels of intratesticular testosterone. Whether this abrupt increase of intratesticular testosterone is specific for cryptorchid testes, or occurs in normal boys as well is not known. Studies in rats suggest that the biosynthesis of testosterone in pubertal cryptorchid testes is higher than in age matched normal testes.[127,128]

Other *in vitro* studies demonstrate a progressive increase of the number of LH receptors in undescended testis with puberty.[103] But the lack of normal controls hampers any judgment on abnormalities. These data cannot invalidate the findings by the French group,[29,86] which are consistent with most of the histologic observations. Final conclusions regarding the suggested hypogonadotrophic hypogonadism in early to mid-puberty must await further studies.

V. STEROIDOGENESIS IN ADULTHOOD

In cryptorchid patients during infancy, childhood and puberty the basal androgen levels are well accepted to be in the normal range for the specific age group. Older studies claim that this is not true for the cryptorchid adult. Basal androgen levels, either in blood plasma or measured in urinary excretion were found to be lower in many cases, although clinical signs of androgen deficiency were not observed. Very early studies by Engberg[129] stated that adult cryptorchid patients excreted only 50% of the amount of androgen that normal subjects excreted in their urine during a 24-h period. He also observed a significant reduction in the concentration of the androgen dependent acid phosphatase in seminal plasma. Since these measurements were carried out using older androgen bioassay methods, his study was repeated by Raboch and Starka[130] with more recent and sophisticated methods. They confirmed the results by Engberg[129] and found in all of their 22 bilateral cryptorchid patients significantly lower plasma androgen levels and acid phosphastase in semen. Both studies did not find differences between patients who underwent orchidopexy during childhood or puberty and unoperated patients. More recent papers showed less clear results finding fewer or no patients with reduced baseline levels of androgens.[76,131-135] Whereas in the 17 patients studied by Gelli et al.,[136] nine have decreased androgen levels, Leitz et al.[95] found 11 in their group out of 39. Other investigators following 23 bilateral cryptorchid patients who underwent orchidopexy before or during puberty, observed only one patient with low androgen levels.[134] In this patient, both testes were atrophic with abnormally elevated gonadotropins,[134] which could be due to the surgical intervention. The same percentage of endocrine insufficiency was observed by Werder et al.[133] with 2 out of 48 cryptorchid men having reduced androgen levels. All of his patients had undergone orchidopexy before puberty. In eight untreated cryptorchid men, complaining about infertility, Agostini et al.[131] did not show any abnormalities in the 24-h urinary excretion of testosterone, 17-ketosteroids, or estrogens. There are no obvious explanations for this discrepancy. Some studies might have had a selection of their patients, taking them from infertility clinics,[129-131] since the studies following pediatric records observed only a very low incidence of reduced androgen levels in their patient group.[76,133-135] Others might have used methods not as exact as the current ones.[129] The number of patients studied by some investigators is too small to come to a definite conclusion.[131,136,137] Another source of irregularities can be the timing and method of blood collection, which is specified in none of the studies. Since almost all patients in the recent studies have undergone orchidopexy, differences between operated and unoperated patients are impossible to assess, and the fact that orchidopexy has cancelled out differences between cryptorchid and healthy subjects cannot be ruled out.

Histological observations in adult cryptorchid human testes are controversial too (see Chapter 5). Some authors do not see any differences in the Leydig cells of cryptorchid testes compared to the contralateral scrotal or to normal testes,[138] others found in 50% of their biopsy material, multivacuolated Leydig cells with large lipid droplets[139,140] or even degenerating Leydig cells.[114] In contrast to these observations, hyperplasia of the Leydig cells was also noted, with an increase in number and individual cell size.[50,139] Unfortunately, none of the studies correlated histological findings with hormone secretion; therefore, the relevance of these findings is not clear. Biochemical studies can confirm the hyperplasia by demonstrating an increased conversion rate of radioactive labeled progesterone per mg tissue in undescended testes.[101] Since the undescended testis is in general smaller than the scrotal testis and the reduction in size is due to a decreased volume of the tubular compartment, there is a relative increase of the Leydig cell mass. Therefore, the steroidogenic capacity, expressed per testis, could be normal or even reduced. Progesterone, when added to *in vitro* cell cultures of Leydig cells of undescended testes, forms the same metabolites as the ones of scrotal testes, suggesting a normal steroidogenic pattern.[99]

In contrast to this, in rats, not only quantitative but also qualitative changes occurred. Higher concentrations of progesterone and 20-alpha-dihydroprogesterone and lower levels of 17-alpha-hydroxyprogesterone and testosterone were found in the abdominal testis in unilateral cryptorchid rats, indicating a block at the 17-alpha-hydroxylase level (Figure 1).[141-143] The high concentration of progesterone is most likely due to a substrate accumulation at the level of the 17-alpha-hydroxylase enzymes, although increased *in vitro* activity of the cholesterol side chain cleavage enzyme complex has been reported[144] and could also lead to increased progesterone levels. However, *in vivo*, the activity of cholesterol side chain cleavage enzyme complex was found to be significantly lower in the cryptorchid rat testis.[105,145] The cause of the blockade of the 17-alpha-hydroxylase in cryptorchid rat testes is not clear and several mechanisms could be related to it. First, the enzyme is temperature sensitive, which has been reported in experimental cryptorchidism.[49] Second, it is known that low doses of hCG (1 to 10 mg) induce *in vitro* an accumulation of progesterone and 17-alpha-hydroxyprogesterone, caused by impaired activities of the enzymes 17-alpha-hydroxylase and 17-20 desmolase.[146] The same reduction in 17-alpha-hydroxylase activity could be induced by 17-beta estradiol and prevented by addition of the antiestrogen tamoxifen.[57,146] In adult rats, surgically made cryptorchid at birth, the intratesticular content of 17-beta-estradiol is significantly elevated,[147] which is probably not due to increased local production, since the aromatase activity in the abdominal testis is lower than in the scrotal testis.[148] The binding capacity for estradiol, however, is significantly increased.[149-151] Whether the increased estrogen content in cryptorchid testis is responsible for the quantitative and qualitative changes observed in the abdominal testis of rats remains to be established, but cannot be dismissed.

Studies in adult cryptorchid rats resembled the same histological picture as the cryptorchid human testis: Leydig cell hyperplasia with increases in the smooth endoplasmic reticulum and unaltered or decreased testosterone levels in the serum with a blunted response to hCG stimulation *in vivo*.[56,106,109,152] These contradictory results, Leydig cells which histologically appear to possess increased steroidogenic capabilities despite normal or reduced peripheral testosterone levels, can be explained by a block in the steroidogenic pathway. This results in impaired testosterone secretion, which in turn leads to increased LH output. The elevated LH concentration stimulates the Leydig cells, resulting in the morphological changes observed.[109] This concept might be true for a subgroup of the patients, since some cryptorchid patients have elevated LH plasma levels,[95,134-136] whereas others present with normal or even subnormal LH concentration, probably reflecting the heterogeneity of cryptorchidism.

Several observations are in disagreement with this hypothesis. For example, in experimental unilateral cryptorchidism the scrotal testis does not show any signs of hyperstimulation,[106] indicating that local factors are responsible for the Leydig cell hypertrophy.[153] Also, *in vitro* stimulation with high doses of hCG resulted in a greater testosterone response in cryptorchid testis than in normal testis.[56,108,154,155] The reason for increased Leydig cell responsiveness *in vitro* while impaired *in vivo* is not known,[156] but reduced uptake of gonadotropins[107] together with a reduced blood flow in the undescended testis might play a role.[157]

Summarizing the reviewed studies, the issue of whether cryptorchid adult men have altered Leydig cell function remains controversial. The direct measurement of serum testosterone was not able to solve this question. The constant incidence of a number of patients with low testosterone serum levels in view of a majority with normal androgen levels supports the theory of heterogeneity among patients with unexplained cryptorchidism. At the same time, one has to be careful in drawing conclusions from patients who underwent orchidopexy, since surgical interference cannot only cancel out possible differences between cryptorchid and normal testis, but can also lead to impaired testicular function, and, on the extreme, to testicular atrophy. However, even in the few patients exhibiting decreased testosterone levels, no clinical signs of primary hypogonadism are detectable, with the patients having normal male hair distribution and normal libido and potency. Therefore, a peripheral androgen deficiency does not exist. The diminished exocrine function of the testis, which is known to require high intratesticular androgen concentration, might therefore be the only indication of decreased androgen production by the Leydig cells.

At the same time, it is not clear whether the observations of increased estradiol concentrations in undescended rat testes are also true for the human. To our knowledge, this has not been studied. Until further information is available, the possibility of increased estradiol binding in the cryptorchid testis, with an inhibitory effect on testicular steroidogenesis, cannot be discounted (see Chapter 6).

VI. CONCLUSIONS

The morphology and function of the Leydig cell in patients with one or two undescended testes is far from being clear and fully understood. This is, in part, due to the heterogeneity of cryptorchidism, either unilateral or bilateral which can be caused by anatomic malformations, genetic disorders, and inborn errors of metabolism as well as by unexplained factors. The testicular descent can vary to a large extent, and the position of the testis might influence its function. In infants and children, ethical reasons prevent detailed studies with large control groups, whereas in adolescents and adults, research is hampered by the fact that most cryptorchid patients undergo orchidopexy at an earlier age. Data obtained in animal experiments have given many important and new insights, but it remains to be proven that making an animal surgically cryptorchid resembles the disease occurring in cryptorchid patients (see Chapter 2). This is especially true when the surgery is performed in adult animals.

The reviewed evidence shows clearly that in early infancy and in adulthood, more patients with idiopathic cryptorchidism reveal lower basal testosterone levels than a normal male of the corresponding age group. During childhood and early puberty, the testosterone response to a hCG stimulation test is blunted in most cryptorchid boys, but becomes normal after previous treatment with hCG or occurs spontaneously in late puberty. It has also been demonstrated that several enzymes of steroidogenesis are temperature sensitive, with lower activities at higher temperatures. Histological findings revealed damaged Leydig cells in all groups. But despite all of these observations, patients with idiopathic cryptorchidism do not show any clinical signs of androgen deficiency. This is true for all age groups, and casts doubts on the significance of the findings mentioned above. It is known, though, that maintenance of libido and potency can be achieved with androgen levels much lower than normal.

The cause of the Leydig cell impairment is not clear. It can be secondary to the location of the testis in slightly increased temperature. On the other hand, it can also be the only, or at least the major, cause for the undescended testis.

The available information also supports the hypothesis of a discrete and transient "hypogonadotrophic hypogonadism". The diminished ability of the pituitary to secrete LH seems to be present at birth and ends during puberty in most cases. No good explanation has been offered for these observations. The lack of stimulation by LH can lead to the Leydig cell impairment and, thus, cause the testis not to descend. Until further studies, it also cannot be dismissed that both impaired Leydig cell function and the diminished LH secretion are the result of an underlying general disturbance.

REFERENCES

1. **Engle, E. T.,** Experimentally induced descent of the testis in the *Maccaca* monkey by hormones from the anterior pituitary and pregnancy serum. The role of gonadokinetic hormones in pregnancy blood in the normal descent of the testis in man, *Endocrinology,* 16, 513, 1932.
2. **Hamilton, J. B.,** The effects of male hormone upon the descent of the testis, *Anat. Rec.,* 70, 533, 1938.
3. **Rajfer, J. and Walsh, P. C.,** Hormonal regulation of testicular descent: experimental and clinical observations, *J. Urol.,* 118, 985, 1977.

4. **Morris, J. M.**, The syndrome of testicular feminization in male pseudohermaphroditism, *Am. J. Obstet. Gynecol.*, 65, 1192, 1953.
5. **Perez-Palacios, G. and Jaffe, R. B.**, The syndrome of testicular feminization, *Pediatr. Clin. North Am.*, 19, 653, 1972.
6. **Habenicht, U. F. and Neumann, F.**, Hormonal regulation of testicular descent, *Adv. Anat. Embryol. Cell Biol.*, 81, 1, 1983.
7. **Elger, W., Richter, J., and Korte, R.**, Failure to detect androgen dependence of the descensus testiculorum in foetal rabbits, mice and monkeys, in *Maldescendus Testis*, Bierich, J. R., Rager, K., and Rancke, M. B., Eds., Urban & Schwarzenberg, Baltimore, 1977, 187.
8. **Morillo-Cucci, G. and German, J.**, Males with a uterus and Fallopian tubes, a rare disorder of sexual development, *Birth Defects Orig. Artic. Series*, 7, 229, 1971.
9. **Armendares, S., Buentello, L., and Frenk, S.**, Two male sibs with uterus and Fallopian tubes: a rare, probably inherited disorder, *Clin. Genet.*, 4, 291, 1973.
10. **Sloan, W. R. and Walsh, P. C.**, Familial persistent Müellerian duct syndrome, *J. Urol.*, 115, 459, 1976.
11. **Forest, M. G., Sizonenko, P. C., Cathiard, A. H., and Bertrand, J.**, Hypophysogonadal function in humans during the first year of life, *J. Clin. Invest.*, 53, 819, 1974.
12. **Job, J.-C. and Gendrel, D.**, Endocrine aspects of cryptorchidism, *Urol. Clin. North Amer.*, 9, 353, 1982.
13. **Roger, M., Mahoul, K., Toublanc, J. E., Castanier, M., Canlorbe, P., and Job, J.-C.**, Les androgenes plasmatiques cher le garcou de la naissance a l'adolescence, *Ann. Pediatr. (Paris)*, 55, 1817, 1979.
14. **Forest, M. G., Cathiard, A. M., and Bertrand, J. A.**, Evidence of testicular activity in early infancy, *J. Clin. Endocrinol. Metab.*, 37, 148, 1973.
15. **Davidson, S., Brisa, M., Zer, A., and Sade, J.**, Plasma testosterone and beta hCG levels in the first twenty-four hours of life in neonates with cryptorchidism, *Eur. J. Pediatr.*, 136, 87, 1981.
16. **Forest, M. G. and Cathiard, A. H.**, Pattern of plasma testosterone and delta-4 androstenedione in normal newborns: evidence for testicular activity at birth, *J. Clin. Endocrinol. Metab.*, 41, 977, 1975.
17. **Winter, J. S. D., Faiwan, C., Hobson, W. C., Prasad, A. V., and Reyes, F. I.**, Pituitary-gonadal relations in infancy. I. Patterns of serum gonadotropin concentrations from birth to four years of age in man and chimpanzee, *J. Clin. Endocrinol. Metab.*, 40, 545, 1975.
18. **Gendrel, D., Chaussain, J. L., Rogers, M., and Job, J.-C.**, Simultaneous postnatal rise of plasma LH and testosterone in male infants, *J. Pediatr.*, 97, 600, 1980.
19. **Winter, J. S. D., Hughes, I. A., Reyes, F. I., and Faiman, C.**, Pituitary-gonadal relations in infancy. II. Patterns of serum gonadal steroid concentrations in man from birth to two years of age, *J. Clin. Endocrinol. Metab.*, 42, 679, 1976.
20. **Tapanainen, J., Koivisto, M., Huhtaniemi, I., and Viliko, R.**, Effect of gonadotropin-releasing hormone on pituitary-gonadal function of male infants during the first year of life, *J. Clin. Endocrinol. Metab.*, 55, 689, 1982.
21. **Forest, M. G., DePeretti, E., and Bertrand, J.**, Hypothalamic-pituitary-gonadal relationships in man from birth to puberty, *Clin. Endocrinol.*, 5, 551, 1976.
22. **Hammond, G. G., Koivisto, M., Kouvalainen, K., and Viliko, R.**, Serum steroids and pituitary hormones in infants with particular reference to testicular activity, *J. Clin. Endocrinol. Metab.*, 49, 40, 1979.
23. **Hammar, M. and Peterson, F.**, Testosterone production in vitro in human testicular tissue, *Andrologia*, 18, 196, 1986.
24. **Van der Molen, H. J. and Rommerts, F. F. G.**, Testicular steroidogenesis, in *The Testis*, Burger, H. and de Kretser, D., Eds., Raven Press, New York, 1981, 213.
25. **Yanaihara, T. and Troen, P.**, Studies of the human testis. I. Biosynthetic pathways for androgen formation in human testicular tissue in vitro, *J. Clin. Endocrinol.*, 34, 783, 1972.
26. **Gendrel, D., Job, J.-C., and Roger, M.**, Reduced post-natal rise of testosterone in plasma of cryptorchid infants, *Acta Endocrinol.*, 89, 372, 1978.
27. **Facchinetti, F., Bracci, R., Sardelli, S., Vanni, M. G., Bagnoli, F., and Genazzani, A. R.**, Possible testicular 3 beta-hydroxysteroid dehydrogenase deficience in cryptorchid neonates, *Arch. Androl.*, 10, 253, 1983.
28. **Rajfer, J., Handelsman, D. J., Swerdloff, R. S., Hurwitz, R., Kaplan, H., Vandergast, T., and Ehrlich, R. M.**, Hormonal therapy of cryptorchidism. A randomized, double-blind study comparing human chorionic gonadotropin and gonadotropin-releasing hormone, *N. Engl. J. Med.*, 314, 466, 1986.
29. **Gendrel, D., Roger, M., Chaussain, J.-L., Canlorbe, P., and Job, J.-C.**, Correlation of pituitary and testicular responses to stimulation test in cryptorchid children, *Acta Endocrinol.*, 86, 641, 1977.
30. **Vanelli, M., Bernasconi, S., Virdis, R., and Giovannelli, G.**, Gonadotropin response to 3 hours LHRH infusion in cryptorchid (C) and normal (N) children, *Pediatr. Res.*, 15, 88, 1981.
31. **Gendrel, D., Roger, M., and Job, J.-C.**, Plasma gonadotropin and testosterone values in infants with cryptorchidism, *J. Pediatr.*, 97, 217, 1980.
32. **Job, J.-C., Gendrel, D., Safar, A., Roger, M., and Chaussain, J.-L.**, Pituitary LH and FSH and testosterone secretion in infants with undescended testes, *Acta Endocrinol.*, 85, 644, 1977.

33. **Swerdloff, R. S. and Heber, D.**, Endocrine control of testicular function from birth to puberty, in *The Testis*, Burger, H. and de Kretser, D., Eds., Raven Press, New York, 1981, 107.

34. **Anoussakis, C., Alexiou, D., Liakakos, D., and Skopelitis, P.**, hCG stimulation test in prepubertal boys with cryptorchidism, *J. Pediatr.*, 93, 630, 1978.

35. **Cacciari, E., Cicognani, A., Pirazzoli, P., Zappulla, F., Tassoni, P., Bernardi, F., and Salardi, S.**, Hypophyso-gonadal function in the cryptorchid child: differences between unilateral and bilateral cryptorchids, *Acta Endocrinol.*, 83, 182, 1976.

36. **Grant, D. B., Laurance, B. M., Atherden, S. M., and Ryness, J.**, hCG stimulation test in children with abnormal sexual development, *Arch. Dis. Child.*, 51, 596, 1976.

37. **Okuyama, A., Itatani, H., Mizutani, S., Sonoda, T., Aono, T., and Matsumoto, K.**, Pituitary and gonadal function in prepubertal and pubertal cryptorchidism, *Acta Endocrinol.*, 95, 553, 1980.

38. **Saez, J. M. and Bertrand, J.**, Studies on testicular function in children: plasma concentrations of testosterone, dehydroepiandrosterone and its sulfate before and after stimulation with human chorionic gonadotropin (1), *Steroids*, 12, 749, 1968.

39. **Winter, J. S. D., Taraska, S., and Faiman, C.**, The hormonal response to hCG stimulation in male children and adolescents, *J. Clin. Endocrinol.*, 34, 348, 1972.

40. **Inano, H. and Tamaoki, B.-I.**, Effect of experimental bilateral cryptorchidism on testicular enzymes related to androgen formation, *Endocrinology*, 83, 1074, 1968.

41. **Kormano, M., Harkonen, M., and Kontinen, E.**, Effect of experimental cryptorchidism on the histochemically demonstrable dehydrogenase of the rat testis, *Endocrinology*, 74, 44, 1964.

42. **Wisner, J. R. and Gomes, W. R.**, Influence of experimental cryptorchidism on cholesterol side-chain cleavage enzymes and alpha 5-3 beta-hydroxysteroid dehydrogenase activities in rat testes, *Steroids*, 31, 189, 1978.

43. **Wisner, J. R. and Gomes, W. R.**, Influence of incubation temperature on activity of cholesterol side-chain cleavage enzymes and alpha 5-3 beta-hydroxysteroid dehydrogenase in rat testis, *J. Endocrinol.*, 65, 143, 1975.

44. **Farr, J. H., Sikka, S., Xie, H. W., Constantinide, D., and Rajfer, J.**, Impaired testosterone biosynthesis in cryptorchidism, *Fertil. Steril.*, 44, 125, 1985.

45. **Niewenhuis, R. J.**, Effect of cryptorchidism and orchidopexy on 3 beta hydroxysteroid dehydrogenase activity in rat testicles, *Arch. Androl.*, 4, 231, 1985.

46. **Samuels, L. T., Bussmann, L., Matsumoto, K., and Huseby, R. A.**, Organization of androgen biosynthesis in the testis, *J. Steroid Biochem.*, 6, 291, 1975.

47. **Hayashi, H. and Harrison, R. G.**, The development of the interstitial tissue of the human testis, *Fertil. Steril.*, 22, 351, 1971.

48. **Hadziselimovic, F.**, Histology and ultrastructure of normal and cryptorchid testes, in *Cryptorchidism — Management and Implications*, Hadziselimovic, F., Ed., Springer-Verlag, Berlin, 1983, 35.

49. **Hadziselimovic, F. and Herzog, B.**, Development of normal and cryptorchid human testes — an ultrastructural study, in *Maldescendus Testis*, Bierich, J. R., Roger, K., and Ranke, M. B., Eds., Urban & Schwarzenberg, Baltimore, 1977, 39.

50. **Sohval, A. R.**, Histopathology of cryptorchidism, *Am. J. Med.*, 16, 346, 1954.

51. **Hadziselimovic, F., Herzog, B., and Seguchi, H.**, Surgical correction of cryptorchidism at 2 years: electron microscopic and morphometric investigations, *J. Pediatr. Surg.*, 10, 19, 1975.

52. **Hadziselimovic, F., Thommen, L., Girard, J., and Herzog, B.**, The significance of postnatal gonadotropin surge for testicular development in normal and cryptorchid testes, *J. Urol.*, 136, 274, 1986.

53. **Chasalow, F., Marr, H., Haour, F., and Saez, J. M.**, Testicular steroidogenesis after human chorionic gonadotropin desensitization in rats, *J. Biol. Chem.*, 254, 5613, 1979.

54. **Cigorraga, S. B., Sorrell, S., Bator, J., Catt, K. J., and Dufau, M. L.**, Estrogen dependence of a gonadotropin-induced steroidogenic lesion in rat testicular Leydig cells, *J. Clin. Invest.*, 65, 699, 1980.

55. **Cigorraga, S. B., Dufau, M. L., and Catt, K. J.**, Regulation of luteinizing hormone receptors and steroidogenesis in gonadotropin-desensitized Leydig cells, *J. Biol. Chem.*, 253, 4297, 1978.

56. **de Kretser, D. M., Sharpe, R. M., and Swanston, I. A.**, Alterations in steroidogenesis and human chorionic gonadotropin binding in the cryptorchid rat testis, *Endocrinology*, 105, 135, 1979.

57. **Nozu, K., Matsuura, S., Catt, K. J., and Dufau, M. L.**, Modulation of Leydig cell androgen biosynthesis and cytochrome P-450 levels during estrogen treatment and human chorionic gonadotropin-induced desensitization, *J. Biol. Chem.*, 256, 10012, 1981.

58. **O'Shaughnessy, P. J. and Payne, A. H.**, Differential effects of single and repeated administration of gonadotropins on testosterone production and steroidogenic enzymes in Leydig cell populations, *J. Biol. Chem.*, 257, 11503, 1982.

59. **Saez, J. M. and Forest, M.**, Kinetics of human chorionic gonadotropin-induced steroidogenic response of human testis. I. Plasma testosterone: implications for human chorionic gonadotropin stimulation test, *J. Clin. Endocrinol. Metab.*, 49, 278, 1979.

60. **Smals, A. G. H., Pieters, G. F. F. M., Drayer, J. I. M., Benraad, T. J., and Kloppenborg, P. W. C.**, Leydig cell responsiveness to single and repeated human chorionic gonadotropin administration, *J. Clin. Endocrinol. Metab.*, 49, 12, 1979.

61. **Smals, A. G. H., Pieters, G. F. F. M., Lozekoot, D. C., Benraad, T. J., and Kloppenborg, P. W. C.**, Dissociated responses of plasma testosterone and 17-hydroxyprogesterone to single or repeated human chorionic gonadotropin administration in normal men, *J. Clin. Endocrinol. Metab.*, 50, 190, 1980.

62. **Wang, C., Rebar, R. W., Hopper, B. R., and Yen, S. S. C.**, Functional studies of the luteinizing hormone-Leydig cell-androgen axis: exaggerated response in C-18 and C-21 testicular steroids to various modes of luteinizing hormone stimulation, *J. Clin. Endocrinol. Metab.*, 51, 201, 1980.

63. **Bhasin, S. and Swerdloff, R. S.**, Mechanisms of gonadotropin-releasing hormone agonist action in the human male, *Endocrin. Rev.*, 7, 106, 1986.

64. **Spratt, D. I., Finkelstein, J. S., Badger, T. M., Butler, J. P., and Crowley, W. F.**, Bio- and immunoactive luteinizing hormone responses to low doses of gonadotropin-releasing hormone (GnRH): dose-response curves in GnRH deficient men, *J. Clin. Endocrinol. Metab.*, 63, 143, 1986.

65. **Meldrum, D. R., Tsao, Z., Monroe, S. E., Braunstein, G. D., Sladek, J., Lu, J. K. H., Vale, W., Rivier, J., Judd, H. L., and Chang, R. J.**, Stimulation of LH fragments with reduced bioactivity following GnRH agonist administration in women, *J. Clin. Endocrinol. Metab.*, 58, 755, 1984.

66. **Winter, J. S. D. and Faiman, C.**, Pituitary-gonadal relations in male children and adolescents, *Pediatr. Res.*, 6, 126, 1972.

67. **Frasier, S. D., Gafford, F., and Horton, R.**, Plasma androgens in childhood and adolescence, *J. Clin. Endocrinol.*, 29, 1404, 1969.

68. **Forest, M. G., Cathiard, A. M., and Bertrand, J. A.**, Total and unbound testosterone levels in the newborn and in normal and hypogonadal children: use of a sensitive radioimmunoassay for testosterone, *J. Clin. Endocrinol. Metab.*, 36, 1132, 1973.

69. **Forest, M. G.**, Pattern of the response to hCG stimulation in prepubertal cryptorchid boys, in *Cryptorchidism: Diagnosis and Treatment*, Job, J.-C., Ed., S. Karger, Basel; *Pediatr. Adolesc. Endocrinol.*, 6, 108, 1979.

70. **Forti, G., Facchinetti, F., Sardelli, S., Griselia, G. A., Santoro, S., Bassi, F., and Serio, M.**, Spermatic and peripheral venous plasma concentrations of progesterone, 17 alpha-hydroxyprogesterone, and 20 alpha-dihydroprogesterone in prepubertal boys, *J. Clin. Endocrinol. Metab.*, 56, 831, 1983.

71. **Illig, R., Torresani, T., Bucher, H., Zachmann, M., and Prader, A.**, Effect of intranasal LHRH therapy on plasma LH, FSH and testosterone and relation to clinical results in prepubertal boys with cryptorchidism, *Clin. Endocrinol.*, 12, 91, 1980.

72. **Rivarola, M. A., Bergada, C., and Cullen, M.**, hCG stimulation test in prepubertal boys with cryptorchidism in bilateral anorchia and in male pseudohermaphroditism, *J. Clin. Endocrinol.*, 31, 256, 1970.

73. **Tapanainen, J., Martikainen, H., Dunkel, L., Perheentupa, J., and Vihko, R.**, Steroidogenic response to a single injection of hCG in pre- and early pubertal cryptorchid boys, *Clin. Endocrinol.*, 18, 355, 1983.

74. **Skorodok, L. M., Savchenko, O. N., Kogan, M. E., and Krasnitskaya, L. N.**, Androgen function of the testes and gonadotropic activity of the pituitary in various forms of cryptorchidism in young boys and adolescents, *Neuro. Sci. Behav. Physiol.*, 12, 489, 1982.

75. **Walsh, P. C., Curry, N., Mills, R. C., and Siiteri, P. K.**, Plasma androgen response to hCG stimulation in prepubertal boys with hypospadias and cryptorchidism, *J. Clin. Endocrinol. Metab.*, 42, 52, 1976.

76. **Koch, H. and Rahlf, G.**, Endocrinologic and morphologic investigations in 208 prepubertal, pubertal or postpubertal patients with cryptorchidism, *Acta Endocrinol. (Kbh.)*, 193 (Suppl.), 85, 1975.

77. **Attanasio, A., Jendricke, U., Bierich, J. R., and Gupta, D.**, Clinical and hormonal effect of human chorionic gonadotropin in prepubertal cryptorchid boys, *J. Endocrinol.*, 63, 50P, 1974.

78. **Gendrel, D., Job, J.-C., Chaussain, J. L., Roger, M., Garnier, P., and Canlorbe, D.**, Pituitary and gonadal responses to stimulation tests in cryptorchid children, in *Cryptorchidism — Diagnosis and Treatment*, Job, J.-C., Ed., S. Karger, Basel; *Pediatr. Adolesc. Endocrinol.*, 6, 121, 1979.

79. **D'Agata, R., Munao, F., and Polosa, P.**, Endocrine function in prepubertal cryptorchids, in *Cryptorchidism*, Bierich, J. R. and Giarola, A., Eds., Academic Press, London, 1979, 225.

80. **Jacobelli, A., Agostino, A., Vecci, E., Simeoni, A., and Ferrantelli, M.**, Studies on the pituitary-testicular axis in boys with cryptorchidism, in *Cryptorchidism*, Bierich, J. R. and Giarola, A., Eds., Academic Press, London, 1979, 261.

81. **Mazzi, C., Riva, L. P., Morandi, G., Mainini, E., Scarsi, G., and Salaroli, A.**, A study of cryptorchid subjects. I. Evaluation of the hypophyseal-testicular axis in the prepuberal period, in *Cryptorchidism*, Bierich, J. R. and Giarola, A., Eds., Academic Press, London, 1979, 269.

82. **Bartolini, E., Galli, P., DelGenevese, A., Panichi, A., Barletta, D., Valicenti, A., Silvestri, D., and Tronchetti, F.**, Pituitary response to constant infusion of LHRH in cryptorchid boys, in *Cryptorchidism*, Bierich, J. R. and Giarola, A., Eds., Academic Press, London, 1979, 351.

83. **Waaler, P. E.**, Endocrinological studies in undescended testes, *Acta Pediatr. Scand.*, 65, 559, 1976.

84. **Dunkel, L., Perheentupa, J., and Apter, D.,** Kinetics of the steroidogenic response to single versus repeated doses of human chorionic gonadotropin in boys in prepuberty and early puberty, *Pediatr. Res.,* 19, 1, 1985.

85. **Hafez, E. S. E., Ghaly, I. M., Ibrahim, I. I., El-Rouby, O., Abdalla, M. I., and Bayad, M. A.,** Endocrine profiles in pediatric andrology. III. Human chorionic gonadotropin stimulation test in cryptorchid boys, *Arch. Androl.,* 11, 53, 1983.

86. **Canlorbe, P., Toublanc, J.-E., Roger, M., and Job, J.-C.,** Etude de la fonction endocrine dans 125 cas de cryptorchidies, *Ann. Med. Interne,* 125, 365, 1974.

87. **Canlorbe, P., Toublanc, J.-E., Job, J.-C., Scholler, R., Roger, M., Castanier, M., and Leymarie, P.,** La fonction endocrine du testicule chez l'enfant ei l'adolescent, *Ann. Pediatr. (Paris),* 21, 13, 1974.

88. **Forest, M. G., David, M., Lecoq, A., Jeune, N., and Bertrans, J.,** Kinetics of the hCG-induced steroidogenic response of the human testis. III. Studies in children of the plasma levels of testosterone and hCG: rationale for testicular stimulation test, *Pediatr. Res.,* 14, 819, 1980.

89. **Scholler, R., Roger, M., Leymarie, P., Castanier, M., Toublanc, J.-E., Canlorbe, P., and Job, J.-C.,** Evaluation of Leydig cell function in normal prepubertal and pubertal boys, *J. Steroid. Biochem.,* 6, 95, 1975.

90. **Sizonenko, P. C., Cuendet, A., and Paunier, L.,** FSH. I. Evidence for its mediating role on testosterone secretion in cryptorchidism, *J. Clin. Endocrinol. Metab.,* 37, 68, 1973.

91. **Marshall, W. A. and Tanner, J. M.,** Variations in the pattern of pubertal changes in boys, *Arch. Dis. Child.,* 45, 13, 1970.

92. **Visser, H. U. A. and Degenhart, H. J.,** Excretion of six individual 17-ketosteroids and testosterone in four girls with precocious sexual hair (premature adrenarche), *Helv. Paediatr. Acta,* 5, 409, 1966.

93. **Rosenfield, R. L.,** Plasma 17-ketosteroids and 17-beta hydroxysteroids in girls with premature development of sexual hair, *J. Pediatr.,* 79, 260, 1971.

94. **Odell, W. D., Swerdloff, R. S., Brain, J., Wollesen, F., and Grover, P. U.,** The effect of sexual maturation on testicular response to LH stimulation of testosterone secretion in the intact rat, *Endocrinology,* 95, 1380, 1974.

95. **Leitz, R., Adam, W., Flach, A., Feder, H., Zwissler, H., Rager, K., Attanasio, A., and Eichner, M.,** Investigations on the hypophyseal-gonadal axis in adults having cryptorchidism in childhood, in *Maldescendus Testis,* Bierich, J. R., Rager, K., and Ranke, M. B., Eds., Urban & Schwarzenberg, Baltimore, 1977, 145.

96. **Laron, Z. and Zilka, E.,** Compensatory hypertrophy of testicle in unilateral cryptorchidism, *J. Clin. Endocrinol.,* 29, 1409, 1969.

97. **Attanasio, A., Rager, U., and Gupta, D.,** Effect of long term hCG administration on plasma androgens in prepubertal cryptorchid boys, in *Maldescendus Testis,* Bierich, J. R., Rager, K., and Ranke, M. B., Eds., Urban & Schwarzenberg, Baltimore, 1977, 125.

98. **Cacciari, E., Cicognani, A., Tassori, P., Flamigni, P., Bolelli, F., Pirazzoli, P., and Salardi, S.,** Plasma testosterone and estradiol concentration in prepubertal boys with cryptorchidism before and after dexamethasone and after human chorionic gonadotropin administration, *Helv. Paediatr. Acta,* 29, 27, 1974.

99. **Berg, A., Lackgren, G., and Lundkvist, U.,** Androgen biosynthesis in cryptorchid and non-cryptorchid human testicular tissue, in *Cryptorchidism,* Bierich, J. R. and Giarola, A., Eds., Academic Press, London, 1979, 231.

100. **Berg, A. A., Kjessler, B., and Lundkvist, U.,** In vitro metabolism of ^{3}H-progesterone in human testicular tissue. II. Prepubertal and adolescent boys, *Acta Endocrinol. (Suppl.),* 207, 23, 1976.

101. **Lackgren, G. and Bergh, A. A.,** In vitro metabolism of progesterone by the human undescended testis, *Int. J. Androl.,* 6, 423, 1983.

102. **Lloyd, J. W., Stecker, J. F., and Rakestraw, M. G.,** In vitro stimulation of adenosine 3',5'-monophosphate in unilateral undescended testes of humans by follicle-stimulating hormone and luteinizing hormone, *J. Clin. Endocrinol. Metab.,* 46, 158, 1978.

103. **Lackgren, G., Ploen, L., Berg, A. A., and Hansson, V.,** Receptors for luteinizing hormone (LH) and follicle-stimulating hormone (FSH) in the human undescended testis and the effect of hCG treatment, *Int. J. Androl.,* 6, 520, 1983.

104. **Bergh, A., Nikula, H., Damber, J. E., Clayton, R., and Huhtaniemi, I.,** Altered concentrations of gonadotropin, prolactin and GnRH receptors, and endogenous steroids in the abdominal testes of adult unilaterally cryptorchid rats, *J. Reprod. Fertil.,* 74, 279, 1985.

105. **Huhtaniemi, I., Bergh, A., Mikula, H., and Damber, J. E.,** Differences in the regulation of steroidogenesis and tropic hormone receptors between the scrotal and abdominal testes of unilaterally cryptorchid adult rats, *Endocrinology,* 115, 550, 1984.

106. **Risbridger, G. P., Kerr, J. B., and de Kretser, D. M.,** Evaluation of Leydig cell function and gonadotropin binding in unilateral and bilateral cryptorchidism: evidence for local control of Leydig cell function by the seminiferous tubules, *Biol. Reprod.,* 24, 534, 1981.

107. **Sharpe, R. M.,** Impaired gonadotropin uptake in vivo by the cryptorchid rat testis, *J. Reprod. Fertil.,* 67, 379, 1983.
108. **Schanbacher, B. D.,** Androgen secretion and characteristics of testicular hCG binding in cryptorchid rats, *J. Reprod. Fertil.,* 59, 145, 1980.
109. **Risbridger, G. P., Kerr, J. B., Peake, R., Rich, K. A., and de Kretser, D. M.,** Temporal changes in rat Leydig cell function after the induction of bilateral cryptorchidism, *J. Reprod. Fertil.,* 63, 415, 1981.
110. **Catt, K. J., Harwood, J. P., Clayton, R. N., Davies, T. F., Chan, V., Katikinemi, M., Nozu, K., and Dufau, M. L.,** Regulation of peptide hormone receptors and gonadal steroidogenesis, *Rec. Prog. Horm. Res.,* 36, 557, 1980.
111. **Risbridger, G. P., Hodgson, Y. M., and de Kretser, D. M.,** Mechanism of action of gonadotropins on the testis, in *The Testis,* Burger, H. and de Kretser, D. M., Eds., Raven Press, New York, 1981.
112. **Hadziselimovic, F.,** Cryptorchidism — Ultrastructure of normal and cryptorchid testis development, *Adv. Anat. Embryol. Cell Biol.,* 53, 1, 1977.
113. **Bigliardi, E. and Vegni-Talluri, M.,** Electron microscopic study of interstitial cells in cryptorchid human testes. I. Interstitial cells in prepubertal age, *Andrologia,* 14, 276, 1982.
114. **Numanoglu, T., Kokturk, I., and Mutaf, O.,** Light and electron microscopic examinations of undescended testicles, *J. Pediatr. Surg.,* 4, 614, 1969.
115. **Lackgren, G. and Berg, A. A.,** The effect of hCG treatment on in vitro metabolism of progesterone by the human undescended prepubertal testis, *Int. J. Androl.,* 6, 414, 1983.
116. **de Kretser, D. M.,** Changes in the fine structure of the human testicular interstitial cells after treatment with human gonadotropins, *Z. Zellforsch.,* 83, 344, 1967.
117. **Job, J.-C., Garnier, P. E., Chaussain, J.-L., Toublanc, J.-E., and Canlorbe, P.,** Effect of synthetic luteinizing hormone-releasing hormone on the release of gonadotropins in hypophyso-gonadal disorders of children and adolescents, *J. Pediatr.,* 84, 371, 1974.
118. **Gendrel, D., Canlorbe, P., Job, J.-C., Roger, M., and Toublanc, J.-E.,** Endocrine data in cryptorchid children, in *Cryptorchidism,* Bierich, J. R. and Giarola, A., Eds., Academic Press, London, 1979, 175.
119. **Lee, P. A., Jaffe, R. B., and Midgley, A. R.,** Serum gonadotropin, testosterone and prolactin concentrations throughout puberty in boys: a longitudinal study, *J. Clin. Endocrinol. Metab.,* 39, 664, 1974.
120. **Judd, H. L., Parker, D. C., Siler, T. M., and Yen, S. S. C.,** The nocturnal rise of plasma testosterone in pubertal boys, *J. Clin. Endocrinol. Metab.,* 38, 710, 1974.
121. **Dickerman, Z., Topper, E., Dintsman, M., Zer, M., Prager-Lewin, R., Kaufman, H., and Laron, Z.,** Pituitary-gonadal function, pubertal development and sperm counts in cryptorchidism: a longitudinal study, in *Cryptorchidism — Diagnosis and Treatment,* Job, J.-C., Ed., S. Karger, Basel; *Pediatr. Adolesc. Endocrinol.,* 6, 195, 1979.
122. **Raboch, J. and Maly, V.,** Somatometrische Befunde bei Mannern mit Keimdrusenstorungen, *Endokrinologie,* 44, 347, 1963.
123. **De la Balze, F. A., Miancini, R. A., Arrillage, F., Andrada, J. A., Vilar, O., Gurtman, A. I., and Davidson, O. W.,** Histologic study of the undescended human testis during puberty, *J. Clin. Endocrinol.,* 20, 286, 1960.
124. **Baccetti, B., Bigliardi, E., Vegni-Talluri, M., Soldani, D., Renieri, T., Selmi, M. G., De Uiartino, A., Bracci, R., and Vanni, M. G.,** The fine structure of the testis in the cryptorchid man, in *Cryptorchidism,* Bierich, J. R. and Giarola, A., Eds., Academic Press, London, 1979, 91.
125. **Houssa, S., de Pape, J., Diebold, N., Feingold, J., and Nezelof, C.,** Cryptorchidism, in *Cryptorchidism — Diagnosis and Treatment,* Job, J.-C., Ed., S. Karger, Basel; *Pediatr. Adolesc. Endocrinol.,* 6, 14, 1979.
126. **Pasqualini, T., Chemes, H., and Rivarola, M. A.,** Testicular testosterone levels during puberty in cryptorchidism, *Clin. Endocrinol.,* 15, 545, 1981.
127. **Gupta, D.,** Endocrinological data in experimental cryptorchidism in the rat, in *Cryptorchidism — Diagnosis and Treatment,* Job, J.-C., Ed., S. Karger, Basel; *Pediatr. Adolesc. Endocrinol.,* 6, 64, 1979.
128. **Rager, U., Arnold, E., Hauschild, A., and Gupta, D.,** Effect of bilateral cryptorchidism on the in vitro transformation of progesterone by testicular tissue at different stages of sexual maturation, *J. Steroid. Biochem.,* 6, 1537, 1975.
129. **Engberg, H.,** Investigations on the endocrine function of the testicle in cryptorchidism, *Proc. R. Soc. Med.,* 42, 652, 1949.
130. **Raboch, J. and Starka, L.,** Plasmatic testosterone in bilateral cryptorchids in adult age, *Andrologie,* 4, 107, 1972.
131. **Agostini, G., Della Morte, E., Felcher, M. L., Gianola, A., and Rolandi, L.,** The dynamic test with GnRH in secondary hypogonadotropic hypogonadism, in *Cryptorchidism,* Bierich, J. R. and Giarola, A., Eds., Academic Press, London, 1979, 345.
132. **Koch, H., Rahlf, G., V. Z. Muhlen, A., Kobberling, J., and Wendenberg, H. J.,** Endokrinologische und morphologiscle Untersuchungen beim Maldescensus testis, *Dtsche. Med. Wochenschr.,* 100, 683, 1975.
133. **Werder, E. A., Illig, R., Tortesani, T., Zachwann, M., Baum, P., Ott, F., and Prader, A.,** Gonadal function in young adults after surgical treatment of cryptorchidism, *Br. Med. J.,* 2, 1357, 1976.

134. **Bramble, F. J., Eccles, S., Houghton, A. L., O'Shea, A., and Jacobs, H. S.**, Reproductive and endocrine function after surgical treatment of bilateral cryptorchidism, *Lancet*, 10, 311, 1974.

135. **Atkinson, P. M., Epstein, M. T., and Rippon, A. E.**, Plasma gonadotropins and androgens in surgically treated cryptorchid patients, *J. Pediatr. Surg.*, 10, 27, 1975.

136. **Gelli, D., Bonomo, M., Ronzoni, M., Loli, P., Colambo, G., Botalla, L., and Silvestrini, F.**, Evaluation of hypophyseal and gonadal function in patients with previous or existing cryptorchidism, in *Cryptorchidism*, Bierich, J. R. and Giarola, A., Eds., Academic Press, London, 1979, 317.

137. **Hedinger, C.**, The histology of the cryptorchid testis, in *Maldescendus Testis*, Bierich, J. R., Rager, K., and Ranke, M. B., Eds., Urban & Schwarzenberg, Baltimore, 1977, 29.

138. **Mancini, R. E., Rosenberg, E., Cullen, M., Lavier, J. C., Vilar, O., Bergada, C., and Andrada, J. A.**, Cryptorchid and scrotal human testis. I. Cryptological, cytochemical and quantitative studies, *J. Clin. Endocrinol.*, 25, 927, 1965.

139. **Hedinger, C.**, Histopathology of the cryptorchid testis, in *Cryptorchidism*, Bierich, J. R. and Giarola, A., Eds., Academic Press, London, 1979, 29.

140. **Nistal, M., Paniagua, R., and Abaurrea, M. A.**, Multi-vacuolated Leydig cells in human adult cryptorchid testes, *Andrologia*, 13, 436, 1981.

141. **Bergh, A., Ason Berg, A., Damber, J. E., Hammar, M., and Selstam, G.**, Steroid biosynthesis and Leydig cell morphology in adult unilaterally cryptorchid rats, *Acta Endocrinol.*, 107, 556, 1984.

142. **Llaurado, J. G. and Dominguez, O. V.**, Effect of cryptorchidism on testicular enzymes involved in androgen biosynthesis, *Endocrinology*, 72, 292, 1963.

143. **Appell, R. A.**, Effect of experimental bilateral cryptorchidism on in vitro metabolism of progesterone by rat testis, *Arch. Androl.*, 7, 79, 1981.

144. **Rommerts, F. F. G., de Jong, F. H., Grootegold, J. A., and van der Molen, H. J.**, Metabolic changes in testicular cells from rats after long-term exposure to 37°C in vivo or in vitro, *J. Endocrinol.*, 85, 471, 1980.

145. **Ficher, M. and Steinberger, E.**, Conversion of progesterone by testicular tissue of cryptorchid rats, *Acta Endocrinol.*, 101, 301, 1982.

146. **Nozu, K., Dehejia, A., Zawistowich, L., Catt, K. J., and Dufau, M. L.**, Gonadotropin-induced receptor regulation and steroidogenic lesions in cultured Leydig cells, *J. Biol. Chem.*, 256, 12875, 1981.

147. **Damber, J. E. and Bergh, A.**, Decreased testicular response to acute LH stimulation and increased intratesticular concentration of oestradiol-17 beta in the abdominal testes in cryptorchid rats, *Acta Endocrinol.*, 95, 416, 1980.

148. **Damber, J. E., Bergh, A., Selstram, G., and Sodergard, R.**, Estrogen receptor and aromatase activity in the testes of the unilateral cryptorchid rat, *Arch. Androl.*, 11, 259, 1983.

149. **Abney, T. O., Grier, H., and Mahesh, V. B.**, Estradiol binding capacity in the cryptorchid rat testis, *Endocrinology*, 101, 975, 1977.

150. **Keel, B. A. and Abney, T. O.**, Alterations of testicular function in the unilaterally cryptorchid rat, *Proc. Soc. Exper. Biol. Med.*, 166, 489, 1981.

151. **Keel, B. A. and Abney, T. O.**, Influence of bilateral cryptorchidism in the mature rat: alterations in testicular function and serum hormone levels, *Endocrinology*, 107, 1226, 1980.

152. **Kerr, J. B., Rich, U. A., and de Kretser, D. M.**, Alterations of the fine structure and androgen secretion of the interstitial cells in the experimental cryptorchid rat testis, *Biol. Reprod.*, 20, 409, 1979.

153. **Wilton, L. J. and de Kretser, D. M.**, The influence of luteinizing hormone on the Leydig cells of cryptorchid rat testes, *Acta Endocrinol.*, 107, 110, 1984.

154. **Hodgson, Y. M. and de Kretser, D. M.**, Testosterone response of cryptorchid and hypophysectomized rats to human chorionic gonadotropin (hCG) stimulation, *Aust. J. Biol. Sci.*, 38, 445, 1985.

155. **Jegou, B., Peake, R. A., Irby, D. C., and de Kretser, D. M.**, Effects of the induction of experimental cryptorchidism and subsequent orchidopexy on testicular function in immature rats, *Biol. Reprod.*, 30, 179, 1984.

156. **Sharpe, R. M., Cooper, I., and Doogan, D. G.**, Increase in Leydig cell responsiveness in the unilaterally cryptorchid rat testis and its relationship to the intratesticular levels of testosterone, *J. Endocrinol.*, 102, 319, 1984.

157. **Damber, J. E., Bergh, A., and Dachlin, L.**, Testicular blood flow, vascular permeability and testosterone production after stimulation of unilaterally cryptorchid adult rats with human chorionic gonadotropin, *Endocrinology*, 117, 1906, 1985.

Chapter 4

TESTICULAR REGULATION OF GONADOTROPIN MICROHETEROGENEITY: EFFECTS OF CRYPTORCHIDISM

Bruce D. Schanbacher, H. Edward Grotjan, Jr., and Brooks A. Keel

TABLE OF CONTENTS

I. INTRODUCTION

Cryptorchidism is an anomaly in mammalian species in which one or both testicles fail to descend into the scrotum.[1] Unilateral and bilateral forms of the anomaly have been reported in humans with sterility observed in 77 and 100% of individuals affected, respectively.[2] While less than 2% of the human male population is naturally affected,[3] cryptorchidism has been imposed experimentally in a variety of species to investigate the pathology of this disorder, including the incidence of neoplasms and dysfunctions within the germinal epithelial and interstitial compartments of the abdominal testis, and to evaluate the acute and chronic responses of these affected individuals to hormonal therapy[4,5] and surgical repair, i.e., orchidopexy.[6] This review on pituitary function in cryptorchid individuals, the feedback regulation of gonadotropin secretion by the abdominal testes, and pituitary gonadotropin microheterogeneity in cryptorchid individuals was prepared to complement the accompanying chapters of this book.

Serum levels of luteinizing hormone (LH), follicle-stimulating hormone (FSH), and testosterone are unaffected in unilaterally cryptorchid rats[7,8] suggesting that the eutopic scrotal testis compensates to overcome the ill-fated endocrine and exocrine functions of its epsilateral, abdominal partner. Atrophic changes are observed in the abdominal testis, whereas the scrotal testis hypertrophies and secretes more testosterone. In contrast to that of unilateral cryptorchids, most studies show that bilateral cryptorchid rats have elevated LH and FSH with little or no change in serum testosterone.[7,9-11] Pronounced elevations in FSH and subtle increases in LH without concomitant changes in testosterone implicate a tubular factor in the normal regulation of pituitary gonadotropin secretion in the rat. Steroids other than testosterone may play a pivotal role,[12,13] but nonsteroidal factors emanating from the seminiferous epithelium are most surely involved.[14,15] Undoubtedly, the spermatogenic arrest observed in the abdominal testes must affect intratesticular communication and endocrine communication between the gonad and the hypothalamo-pituitary system.

II. THE GONADOTROPES

In both castrate and cryptorchid rats, pituitary production of LH and particularly FSH are increased (Table 1) causing typical "castration cells" to appear in the adenohypophysis. The existence of two kinds of gonadotropic cells was suggested as early as 1954 in the pioneering studies of Farquhar and Rinehart.[16] In general, LH-secreting cells have a small cell body while FSH-secreting cells are larger. In many cases both cell types are located along blood capillaries dispersed throughout the adenohypophysis, but they are most numerous either in the central portion of the lateral lobes or in a superficial area adjacent to the neurohypophysis. Both gonadotropes have eccentric, sometimes indented nuclei, well-developed Golgi apparatuses, as well as abundant rough endoplasmic reticuli and secretory granules. In castrate and cryptorchid cells, the rough endoplasmic reticulum of FSH secreting cells is noticeably hypertrophied. In view of the relative hypersecretion of FSH in cryptorchids and associated increase in FSH/LH secretory ratio, it is interesting to note that immunocytochemical assessment has led some investigators to conclude that LH and FSH may be secreted by the same gonadotrope.[17]

The relationship between the endocrine products of the testes and the secretory activity of the adenohypophysis is incompletely understood, particularly in the cryptorchid male. In rats,[9] sheep,[18] cattle,[19] horses,[20] rhesus macaques,[21] and men,[22] cryptorchidism results in elevated circulating levels of LH and FSH demonstrating an altered feedback relationship between testicular secretions and the pituitary gonadotropes. Experimentally induced bilateral cryptorchidism in several nonhuman species causes blood gonadotropin levels to rise in the absence of a change in circulating testosterone.[7,12,21,23,24] In contrast, gonadotropin increases are not always observed in the cryptorchid child,[25,26] but exceptions have been reported.[22]

Table 1

EFFECTS OF CRYPTORCHIDISM ON SERUM LH CONCENTRATIONS AND PITUITARY LH AND FSH CONTENT IN MALE RATS AND RAMS[52]

	Rats		Rams				
	Serum LH	Pituitary LH	Serum LH	Pituitary LH		Pituitary FSH	
Treatment	(ng/ml)	(µg)	(ng/ml)	(µg/mg)	(µg)	(µg/100 mg)	(µg)
Intact	0.73 ± 0.14[a]	1.34 ± 0.03[a]	0.23 ± 0.06[a]	0.96 ± 0.13[a]	470 ± 60[a]	3.94 ± 0.77[a]	18.32 ± 2.23[a]
Cryptorchid	2.15 ± 0.40[b]	2.42 ± 0.21[b]	3.34 ± 1.56[b]	1.32 ± 0.21[a]	796 ± 98[b]	10.53 ± 1.20[b]	64.58 ± 7.00[b]

Note: Values with the same superscript letters are not significantly different ($p > 0.05$) by Student t test.

[a,b] Mean ± SEM for six to eight rats and five rams per group.

Intravenous and intranasal challenge with luteinizing hormone releasing hormone (LHRH) or its analogs have been used to treat cryptorchid individuals as an alternative to orchidopexy,[27] and have served as useful diagnostic tools for the assessment of pituitary function and gonadotropin reserve.[22] Serum testosterone levels are not affected by testis position in boys, yet basal and LHRH-induced gonadotropin release are significantly elevated in bilateral cryptorchid boys when compared to normal or unilateral cryptorchid boys;[22] the difference being more pronounced for FSH than for LH. Similar findings suggest that endogenous testosterone participates in a somewhat secondary role to control pituitary gonadotropin secretion and that the germinal elements within the seminiferous tubules exert a more pronounced regulatory effect on the pituitary, particularly on FSH-secreting cells. Elevated serum LH following cryptorchidism is indicative of hypofunction not only of the seminiferous tubules but also of Leydig cells within the ectopic (abdominal) testis.[28-30] Alternatively, blunted testosterone secretion in postnatal cryptorchid boys has been attributed to a primary LH defect.[31]

III. GONADOTROPIN MICROHETEROGENEITY

The pituitary gonadotropins LH and FSH are composed of a common alpha subunit and a hormone-specific beta subunit.[32] The subunits of the respective hormones are synthesized individually and subsequently combined to form the alpha-beta dimers found in the native hormone. The alpha subunit of several species is produced in excess,[33-36] but the physiological role of the uncombined subunit remains unclear.

The pituitary gonadotropins also exhibit charge microheterogeneity and thus exist as a series of isohormones with different net charges or isoelectric points.[37-41] These isohormones also differ with respect to receptor binding activities[42] and biological potencies.[40,43,44] Especially pertinent to this discussion is the observation that reproductive status, including both castration[38,45-47] and cryptorchidism,[48] alters both the quality and quantity of LH produced by the pituitary. Undoubtedly, pituitary synthesis of gonadotropins is under hormonal control and production of the most active biological forms of these hormones is influenced by the steroid environment in which they are produced.[47,49] Using this scenario, it would seem reasonable to conclude that changes in testicular secretions could be self directing by acting at the level of the pituitary to change not only the quantity but also the quality of gonadotropins being produced and secreted.

The increase in circulating gonadotropin following experimentally induced cryptorchidism is based on the imprecise results of hormone radioimmunoassay. These assays often utilize antisera with different specificities, thus it is difficult to equate the results from different laboratories and to be assured that differences in the various immunoreactive forms of the respective gonadotropins do not occur in response to cryptorchidism. The possibility that cryptorchidism and associated changes in testicular steroid environment may affect the secreted isoforms of either LH or FSH is suspected but remains unproven at present. The following discussion presents preliminary data on the relative amounts of LH and FSH isohormones in the pituitary of cryptorchid rats and rams.

A. Luteinizing Hormone (LH)

Figure 1 compares the elution profiles of immunoreactive LH in pituitary extracts of intact and castrate male rats chromatofocused on pH 10.5 to 7.0 gradients.[46] Seven isohormones of rLH were identified and designated isohormones I through VII. Note the relative abundance of isohormone I in the elution profile of intact rats and its relative absence in castrate rats. Not only were the same seven isohormones identified in another study with rats[48] but the immunoreactive form eluted as isohormone I (elution pH >9.8) was even more prevalent in extracts of bilateral cryptorchid rats (Figure 2). For comparison, the results of these two

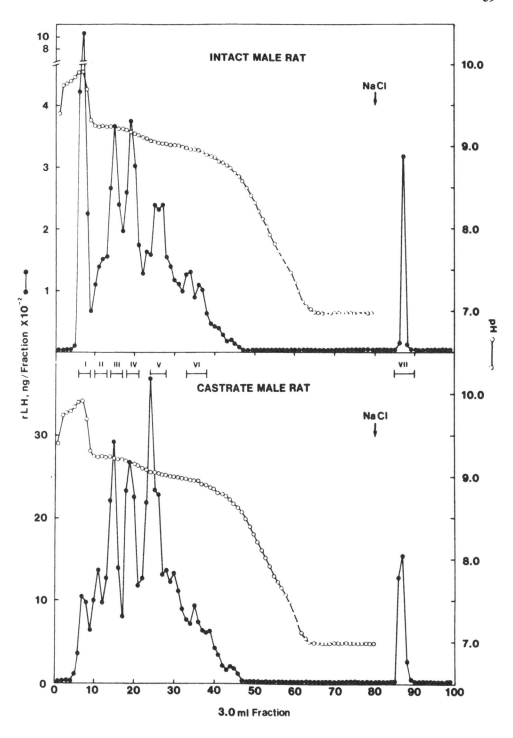

FIGURE 1. Chromatofocusing elution profiles of immunoreactive rLH in the extracts of anterior pituitaries from intact (top) and castrate (bottom) male rats. Each profile represents the mean obtained from three separate chromatofocusing profiles; an extract of four pituitaries was used in each determination. Note that the ordinate scale for castrates is tenfold larger than that for intact rats. Brackets correspond to the fractions pooled to divide the elution profiles into isohormones, which are designated with Roman numerals. Peak I (elution pH >9.8) elutes before the gradient starts to form, and peak VII (elution pH <7.0) elutes only after treatment of the column with 1.0 M NaCl (arrow). (From Keel, B. A. and Grotjan, H. E., Jr., *Endocrinology*, 117, 354, 1985. With permission.)

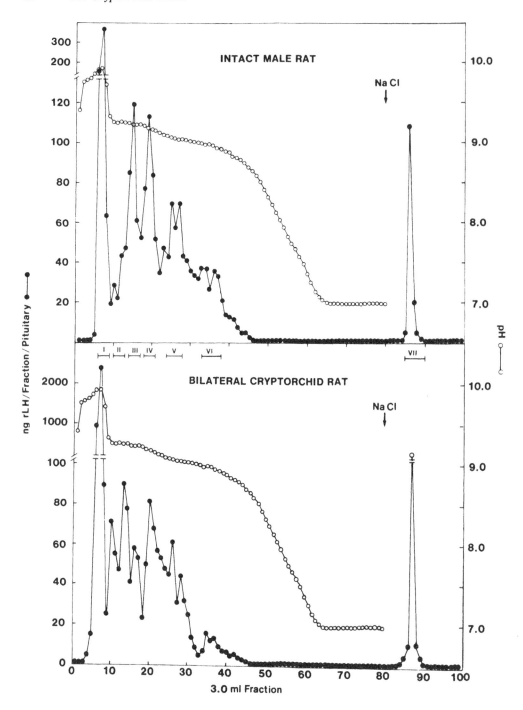

FIGURE 2.   Chromatofocusing elution profiles of immunoreactive rLH in the extracts of pituitaries from intact male (top) and bilaterally cryptorchid (bottom) rats. Data are expressed as the mean ng rLH per fraction per pituitary (n = 2). Brackets correspond to the fractions pooled to divide the profiles into respective isohormones, which are designated by Roman numerals. Peak I (elution pH >9.8) elutes before the gradient starts to form and Peak VII (elution pH <7.0) elutes only after treatment of the column with 1.0 *M* NaCl (arrow). (From Keel, B. A. and Grotjan, H. E., Jr., *Biol. Reprod.*, 32, 83, 1985. With permission.)

studies are presented together in Table 2. Whether expressed in either absolute or relative terms, isohormones III through VI having elution pHs between 9.23 and 8.97 were reduced in cryptorchid rats when compared to intact rats. The biological potencies of these various isohormones were assessed by the in vitro rat interstitial cell bioassay using the same NIH-rLH-15 standard. The biological to immunological (B:I) ratios were clearly related to elution pH and decreased with decreasing elution pH in both intact and cryptorchid rats. The B to I ratios of isohormone I were three- to fourfold higher than those of isohormone VII. The distribution of biologically active LH (termed "bio-index" in Reference 47) shows that isohormone I is the only form affected by cryptorchidism (Figure 3). These findings in the rat demonstrate that cryptorchidism causes both a relative and an absolute change in the various rLH isohormones, with a marked increase in the most active form, i.e., isohormone I. Considering that serum testosterone is normal or slightly below normal in cryptorchid rats and assuming that the LH found in pituitary extracts reflects that normally secreted, it seems reasonable to conclude that both quantitative and qualitative changes in LH secretion are required to achieve adequate stimulation of the abdominal testis in cryptorchid rats.

Ovine pituitary LH also separates into various isohormones during chromatofocusing.[47] Eight isohormones with elution pHs greater than have been identified in male sheep. This is shown graphically in Figures 4 and 5 for castrate and cryptorchid rams, respectively, compared to their intact counterparts. The castration and cryptorchidism studies were done at different times of the year and on different age animals. In rams, about half of the immunoreactive LH was recovered in peaks F and G having elution pHs of 8.91 and 8.81, respectively. Castration and cryptorchidism resulted in a subtle shift toward more basic forms of the hormone. Cryptorchid rams had a smaller percentage of oLH in peak F with a corresponding increase in peaks D and E. The distribution of immunoreactive LH isohormones is shown for intact, castrate, and cryptorchid rams in Table 3.

In summary, the endocrine changes associated with bilateral cryptorchidism induce subtle changes in pituitary LH microheterogeneity. The only significant effect was seen in the rat wherein the most basic form of LH (isohormone A, pI >9.8) was increased by cryptorchidism. A more subtle change was observed in cryptorchid rams. Because testicular steroids have been shown to substantially alter the distribution of immunoreactive LH isohormones in castrate male sheep,[47] it seems reasonable to conclude that testicular steroid secretions are nominally affected by cryptorchidism in this species. If this explanation is accepted, then one must suspect more dramatic changes in steroid secretion by the rat testis when relocated to the abdomen. Interestingly, in these and other species, serum testosterone is generally reported to be in the normal range of values for healthy, intact males. Preliminary data from our laboratories indicate no effect of cryptorchidism on the molecular weight or the concentrations of immunoreactive LH, LH alpha subunit, and LH beta subunit in ovine pituitary extracts.[52]

B. Follicle-Stimulating Hormone (FSH)

Figure 6 compares the FSH immunoreactive elution profiles of intact ram and wether pituitary extracts when chromatofocused on pH 7.5 to 4.0 gradients.[50] When ram pituitary extracts were chromatofocused, at least nine immunoreactive peaks of oFSH were observed. Seven forms focused within the defined limits of the gradient and exhibited reproducible elution pHs ranging from 6.74 to 4.10. These forms were designated as isohormones B through H (Table 4). Two additional forms of oFSH were also observed: one in the void volume of the column (isohormone A; elution pH >7.4) and one which was bound to the column but could be eluted with 1 M NaCl (isohormone Z; elution pH <4.0). Castration resulted in a significant fourfold increase in the relative amounts of isohormone B and a slight increase in isohormone C (Table 4). A slight but significant increase in the relative amount of isohormone Z was also apparent, while isohormones E and H were reduced by

Table 2

RELATIVE AMOUNTS[a] OF rLH ISOHORMONES (SEPARATED BY CHROMATOFOCUSING) IN PITUITARIES OF CASTRATE, INTACT, AND CRYPTORCHID MALE RATS

Isohormone	Elution pH	Study 1		Study 2	
		Castrate	Intact	Intact	Cryptorchid
I	>9.80	7.2 ± 1.1	24.9 ± 7.0	31.3 ± 5.3	71.8 ± 9.3
II	9.25	11.0 ± 1.4	8.8 ± 1.4	7.5 ± 1.0	7.4 ± 2.1
III	9.23	17.4 ± 2.1	16.0 ± 2.4	14.9 ± 3.6	3.8 ± 1.0
IV	9.17	20.1 ± 2.4	17.0 ± 1.8	15.6 ± 2.0	5.7 ± 2.5
V	9.06	25.9 ± 2.7	16.6 ± 3.1	13.7 ± 1.4	4.7 ± 1.9
VI	8.97	10.5 ± 2.3	9.6 ± 1.4	9.5 ± 0.4	1.4 ± 0.1
VII	<7.00	7.7 ± 0.7	6.8 ± 1.4	7.4 ± 2.3	5.0 ± 1.7

[a]   Mean ± SEM (n = 2 or 3) percentage of immunoreactive rLH obtained in each isohormone. For the precise statistical relationships, please refer to References 46 and 48.

Data from Study 1 and Study 2 are from References 46 and 48, respectively.

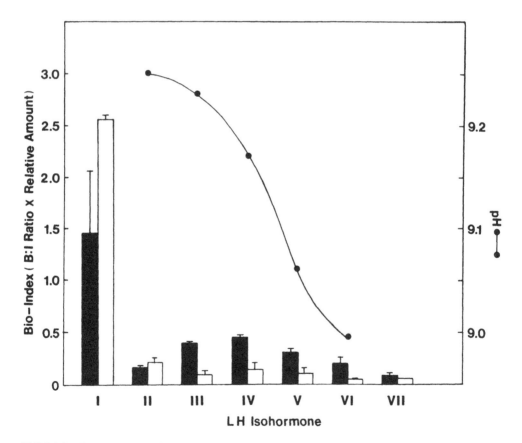

FIGURE 3.   Distribution of biologically active rLH among its isohormones ("bio-index") in intact (solid bars) and bilaterally cryptorchid (open bars) male rats. Elution pHs (●—●) for isohormones II through VI are expressed as the mean of four determinations. Bars identified with the same letter are not significantly different (*p* >0.05) by one-way analysis of variance and Duncan's test. (From Keel, B. A. and Grotjan, H. E., Jr., *Biol. Reprod.*, 32, 83, 1985. With permission.)

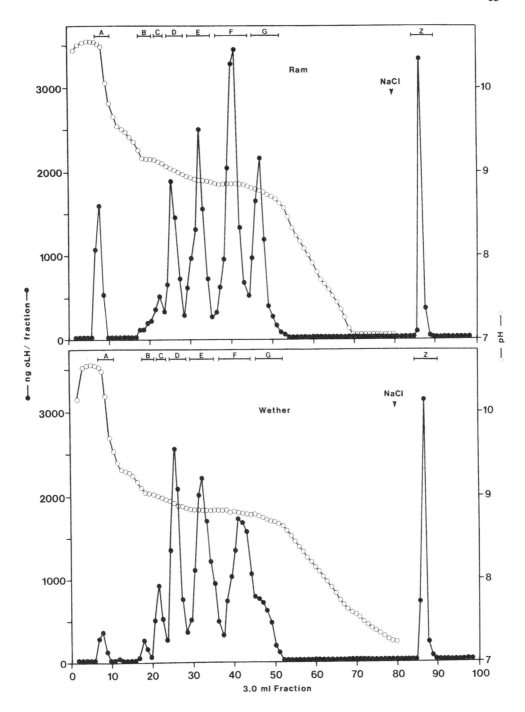

FIGURE 4.   Representative chromatofocusing elution profiles of immunoreactive oLH in the extracts (100,000 × *g* supernatant) of anterior pituitaries from a ram (top) and wether (bottom). Note that isohormone A eluted before the pH gradient started to form (elution pH >9.8) and that isohormone Z bound to the column but eluted with 1.0 *M* NaCl. Brackets correspond to fractions pooled to divide the profiles into respective isohormones. (From Keel, B. A., Schanbacher, B. D., and Grotjan, H. E., Jr., *Biol. Reprod.*, 36, 1102, 1987. With permission.)

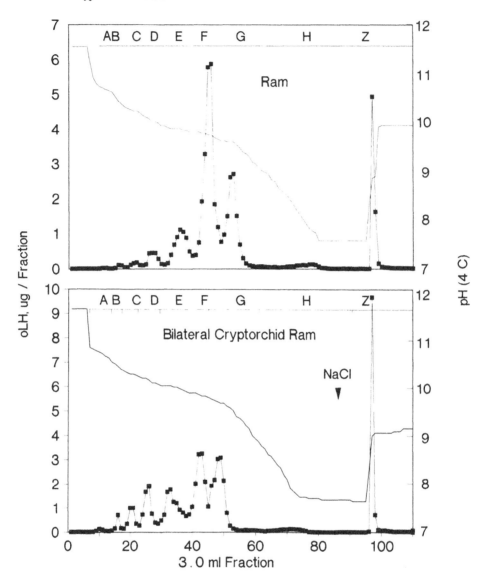

FIGURE 5. Representative chromatofocusing elution profiles of immunoreactive oLH in the extracts (100,000 × *g* supernatant) of anterior pituitaries from an intact (top) and a cryptorchid (bottom) ram. Note that isohormone A eluted before the pH gradient started to form (elution pH >9.8) and that isohormone Z bound to the column but eluted with 1.0 *M* NaCl. Brackets correspond to fractions pooled to divide the profiles into respective isohormones. (From Schanbacher, B. D., Keel, B. A., and Grotjan, H. E., Jr., unpublished data, 1989.)

approximately twofold in wethers. Interestingly, these castration-induced alterations could be reversed by steroid administration,[50] suggesting a role of gonadal steroid feedback regulation in the production of oFSH isohormones. Similar chromatofocusing profiles for pituitary immunoreactive oFSH were also observed in intact and cryptorchid rams (Figure 7). Several cryptorchid ram profiles displayed an apparent increase in the relative amount of isohormone B characteristic of a wether profile. However, statistical analysis failed to reveal any differences between the relative distributions of intact and cryptorchid oFSH (Table 4). With the convincing argument that inhibin participates in the regulation of FSH secretion by the pituitary,[14] it is perhaps surprising that the marked reduction in the testicular inhibin levels associated with cryptorchidism[51] does not affect the distribution of FSH isohormones in cryptorchid rams. To date, no information is available on the possible effects of inhibin on gonadotropin microheterogeneity.

Table 3

RELATIVE AMOUNTS[a] OF oLH ISOHORMONES (SEPARATED BY CHROMATOFOCUSING) IN PITUITARIES OF CASTRATE, INTACT, AND CRYPTORCHID RAMS

Isohormone	Elution pH	Study 1		Study 2	
		Castrate	Intact	Intact	Cryptorchid
A	>9.80	1.5 ± 0.3	2.9 ± 2.4	0.3 ± 0.1	0.5 ± 0.1
B	9.36	2.1 ± 0.3	0.8 ± 0.4	0.7 ± 0.1	1.1 ± 0.2
C	9.19	7.2 ± 0.7	1.8 ± 0.5	1.1 ± 0.2	2.4 ± 0.8
D	9.07	14.9 ± 1.8	6.8 ± 2.6	3.6 ± 0.7	6.6 ± 0.9
E	8.97	25.8 ± 0.9	14.5 ± 3.2	8.5 ± 1.6	14.8 ± 0.7
F	8.88	24.8 ± 0.9	33.7 ± 3.4	42.9 ± 2.2	30.9 ± 2.7
G	8.76	13.8 ± 3.4	23.5 ± 3.5	22.6 ± 1.3	24.2 ± 0.7
H	7.30	—	—	3.0 ± 0.3	2.4 ± 0.3
Z	<7.00	9.9 ± 0.9	15.8 ± 6.9	17.4 ± 2.2	17.1 ± 1.6

[a] Mean ± SEM (n = 5) percentage of immunoreactive oLH obtained in each isohormone. For the precise statistical relationships, please refer to Reference 47.

Data from Study 1 and Study 2 are from References 47 and 52, respectively.

IV. CONCLUSIONS

Bilateral cryptorchidism, like castration, produces a marked increase in the circulating levels of LH and FSH, suggesting that translocation of the testes to an abdominal position upsets the normal feedback balance between the hypothalamus, pituitary and testis. Removal of gonadal feedback moieties by castration alters not only the quantity of pituitary gonadotropins but also critically changes the quality of the hormone by changing the distribution of the hormones' isoelectric variants. This castration-induced alteration of gonadotropin microheterogeneity can markedly affect the overall biological activity of the hormone. In contrast to castration, bilateral cryptorchidism increases circulating levels of gonadotropin without markedly affecting androgen secretion by the testis. The endocrine changes associated with cryptorchidism significantly alter both rat and ovine LH microheterogeneity but these changes are subtle. The effects of bilateral cryptorchidism on the synthesis of pituitary LH and FSH and on the biopotency of the secreted variants of these gonadotropins remain to be examined.

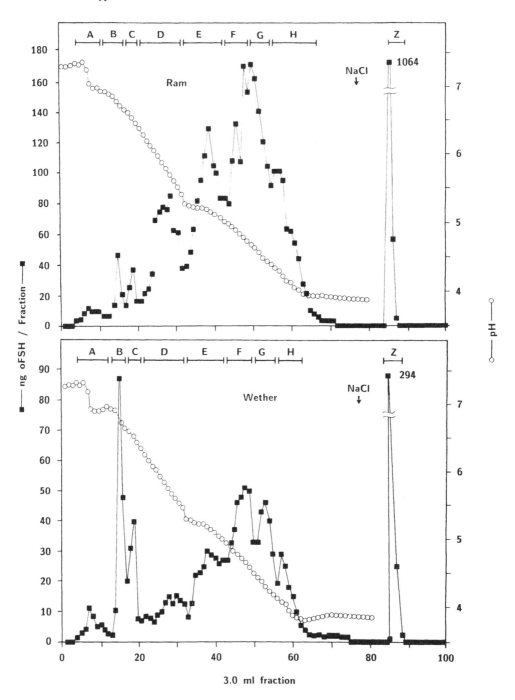

FIGURE 6.   Representative chromatofocusing elution profiles of immunoreactive oFSH in the extracts (100,000 × *g* supernatant) of anterior pituitaries from a ram (top) and a wether (bottom). Note that isohormone A eluted before the pH gradient started to form (elution pH >7.4) and that isohormone Z bound to the column but eluted with 1.0 *M* NaCl. Brackets correspond to fractions pooled to divide the profiles into respective isohormones. (From Keel, B. A. and Schanbacher, B. D., *Biol. Reprod.*, 37, 386, 1987. With permission.)

Table 4
RELATIVE AMOUNTS[a] OF oFSH ISOHORMONES (SEPARATED BY CHROMATOFOCUSING) IN PITUITARIES OF CASTRATE, INTACT, AND CRYPTORCHID RAMS

Isohormone	Elution pH	Study 1		Study 2	
		Castrate	Intact	Intact	Cryptorchid
A	>7.40	4.5 ± 0.8	2.0 ± 0.5	7.6 ± 1.8	4.1 ± 1.0
B	6.74	8.4 ± 1.4	2.2 ± 0.2	5.2 ± 1.4	5.6 ± 1.0
C	6.52	4.3 ± 1.0	2.4 ± 0.5	4.6 ± 0.7	3.2 ± 0.7
D	5.76	7.5 ± 0.7	9.8 ± 1.3	10.1 ± 2.2	7.9 ± 1.3
E	5.20	10.5 ± 1.8	18.1 ± 2.0	13.7 ± 1.1	12.8 ± 0.9
F	4.74	19.2 ± 1.0	17.2 ± 5.2	10.6 ± 1.0	14.6 ± 2.2
G	4.44	10.9 ± 0.8	12.3 ± 1.1	12.1 ± 1.3	11.1 ± 0.9
H	4.10	6.5 ± 1.0	15.8 ± 2.7	17.7 ± 4.8	14.0 ± 2.9
Z	<4.00	28.2 ± 4.0	20.2 ± 4.0	18.3 ± 3.4	27.2 ± 1.1

[a] Mean ± SEM (n = 5) percentage of immunoreactive oFSH obtained in each isohormone. For the precise statistical relationships, please refer to Reference 47.

Data from Study 1 and Study 2 are from References 50 and 52, respectively.

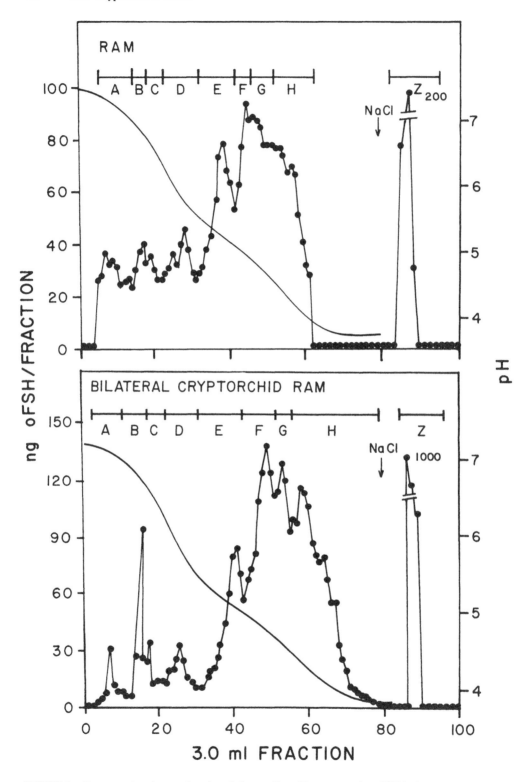

FIGURE 7.   Representative chromatofocusing elution profiles of immunoreactive oFSH in the extracts (100,000 × *g* supernatant) of anterior pituitaries from an intact (top) and a cryptorchid (bottom) ram. Note that isohormone A eluted before the pH gradient started to form (elution pH >7.4) and that isohormone Z bound to the column but eluted with 1.0 *M* NaCl. Brackets correspond to fractions pooled to divide the profiles into respective isohormones. (From Schanbacher, B. D., Keel, B. A., and Grotjan, H. E., Jr., unpublished data, 1989.)

REFERENCES

1. **Hunter, J.,** Observations on the state of the testis in the foetus, and on the hernia congenita, in *Hunter Medical Commentaries,* Part 1, 1962.
2. **Bayle, H.,** Du traitement chirurgical des cryptorchidies; dans la fonction endocrine du testicule, Masson, Paris, 1957.
3. **Moormann, J. G.,** Histochemische Untersuchungen bei der Lageanomalie des Hodens mach Behandlung mit humanen Chorion-Gonadotropin (LCG) im Tierversuch und am Klinischen Kraukengut, *Ann. Univ. Sarav.,* 19, 2, 1972.
4. **Happ, J., Kollmann, F., Krawehl, C., Neubauer, M., Krause, U., Demisch, K., Sandow, J., Rechenberg, W., and Beyer, J.,** Treatment of cryptorchidism with prenasal gonadotropin-releasing hormone therapy, *Fertil. Steril.,* 29, 546, 1978.
5. **Illig, R., Torresani, T., Bucher, H., Zachmann, M., and Prader, A.,** Effect of intranasal LHRH therapy on plasma LH, FSH and testosterone, and relation to clinical results in prepubertal boys with cryptorchidism, *Clin. Endocrinol.,* 12, 91, 1980.
6. **Silber, S.,** Testicular transplantation and autotransplantation, in *Vascular Problems in Urologic Surgery,* Novick, A. C. and Straffon, R. A., Eds., W. B. Saunders, Philadelphia, 1982, 337.
7. **Gomes, W. R. and Jain, S. K.,** Effect of unilateral and bilateral castration and cryptorchidism on serum gonadotrophins in the rat, *J. Endocrinol.,* 68, 191, 1976.
8. **Keel, B. A. and Abney, T. O.,** Alterations of testicular function in the unilaterally cryptorchid rat, *Proc. Soc. Exp. Biol. Med.,* 166, 489, 1981.
9. **Swerdloff, R. S., Walsh, P. C., Jacobs, H. S., and Odell, W. D.,** Serum LH and FSH during sexual maturation in the male rat: effect of castration and cryptorchidism, *Endocrinology,* 88, 120, 1971.
10. **Rager, K., Zarzycki, J., Eichner, M., and Gupta, D.,** Effects of experimental bilateral cryptorchidism and castration on the plasma gonadotropins in male rats during sexual maturation, *Res. Exp. Med.,* 165, 55, 1975.
11. **Bhasin, S., Fielder, T. J., Sod-Moriah, U. A., and Swerdloff, R. S.,** Testicular modulation of luteinizing hormone response to gonadotropin-releasing hormone (GnRH)-agonist treatment, *Biol. Reprod.,* 36, 309, 1987.
12. **Schanbacher, B. D. and Ford, J. J.,** Gonadotropin secretion in cryptorchid and castrate and the acute effects of exogenous steroid treatment, *Endocrinology,* 100, 387, 1979.
13. **Schanbacher, B. D.,** The regulation of FSH secretion in rams, *J. Reprod. Fertil.,* Suppl. 26, 15, 1979.
14. **de Kretser, D. M.,** Inhibin becomes a reality, *Res. Reprod.,* 18, 1, 1986.
15. **Blanc, M. R., Cahoreau, C., Courot, M., Dacheux, J. L., Hochereau-de-Reviers, M. Th., and Pisselet, Cl.,** Plasma follicle stimulating hormone (FSH) and luteinizing hormone (LH) suppression in the cryptorchid ram by a non-steroidal factor (inhibin) from ram rete testis fluid, *Int. J. Androl.,* Suppl. 2, 139, 1978.
16. **Farquhar, M. G. and Rinehart, J. F.,** Electron microscopic studies of the anterior pituitary gland of castrate rats, *Endocrinology,* 54, 516, 1954.
17. **Childs, G. V., Hyde, C., Noar, Z., and Catt, K.,** Heterogeneous luteinizing hormone and follicle stimulating hormone storage patterns in subtypes of gonadotropes separated by centrifugal elutriation, *Endocrinology,* 113, 2120, 1983.
18. **Hillard, M. A. and Bindon, B. M.,** Plasma LH patterns in cryptorchid rams and wethers, *J. Reprod. Fertil.,* 43, 379, 1975.
19. **Schanbacher, B. D.,** Cryptorchidism and the pituitary-testicular axis in bulls, *J. Reprod. Fertil.,* Suppl. 30, 67, 1981.
20. **Schanbacher, B. D. and Pratt, B. R.,** Response of a cryptorchid stallion to vaccination against luteinizing hormone releasing hormone, *Vet. Rec.,* 116, 74, 1985.
21. **Resko, J. A., Jackson, G. L., Huckins, C., Stadelman, H., and Spies, H. G.,** Cryptorchid rhesus macaques: long term studies on changes in gonadotropins and gonadal steroids, *Endocrinology,* 107, 1127, 1980.
22. **Okuyama, A., Itatani, H., Mizutani, S., Sonada, T., Aono, T., and Matsumoto, K.,** Pituitary and gonadal function in prepubertal and pubertal cryptorchidism, *Acta Endocrinol.,* 95, 553, 1980.
23. **Gupta, D., Rager, K., Zarzycki, J., and Eichner, M.,** Levels of luteinizing hormone, follicle stimulating hormone, testosterone and dihydrotestosterone in the circulation of sexually maturing intact male rats and after orchidectomy and experimental bilateral cryptorchidism, *J. Endocrinol.,* 66, 183, 1975.
24. **Schanbacher, B. D.,** Testosterone secretion in cryptorchid and intact bulls injected with gonadotropin-releasing hormone and luteinizing hormone, *Endocrinology,* 104, 360, 1979.
25. **Cacciari, E., Cicognani, A., Pirazzoli, P., Zappulla, F., Tassoni, P., Bernardi, F., and Salardi, S.,** Hypophysio-gonadal function in the cryptorchid child: differences between unilateral and bilateral cryptorchids, *Acta Endocrinol.,* 83, 182, 1976.
26. **Job, J.-C., Gendrel, D., Safar, A., Roger, M., and Chaussain, J.-L.,** Pituitary LH and FSH and testosterone secretion in infants with undescended testes, *Acta Endocrinol.,* 85, 644, 1977.

27. **Illig, R., Torresani, T., Bucher, H., Zachmann, M., and Prader, A.,** Effect of intranasal LHRH therapy on plasma LH, FSH and testosterone, and relation to clinical results in prepubertal boys with cryptorchidism, *Clin. Endocrinol.,* 12, 91, 1980.

28. **de Kretser, D. M., Sharpe, R. M., and Swanston, I. A.,** Alterations in steroidogenesis and human chorionic gonadotropin binding in the cryptorchid rat testis, *Endocrinology,* 105, 135, 1979.

29. **Schanbacher, B. D.,** Androgen response of cryptorchid and intact rams to ovine LH, *J. Reprod. Fertil.,* 59, 151, 1980.

30. **Schanbacher, B. D.,** Gonadotropin secretion and testis function in artificially cryptorchid bulls, *Theriogenology,* 10, 231, 1978.

31. **Gendrel, D., Job, J.-C., and Roger, M.,** Reduced post-natal rise of testosterone in plasma of cryptorchid infants, *Acta Endocrinol.,* 89, 372, 1978.

32. **Pierce, J. G. and Parsons, T. F.,** Glycoprotein hormones: structure and function, *Annu. Rev. Biochem.,* 50, 465, 1981.

33. **Prentice, L. G. and Ryan, R. J.,** LH and its subunits in human pituitary, serum and urine, *J. Clin. Endocrinol. Metab.,* 40, 303, 1975.

34. **Grotjan, H. E., Jr., Leveque, N. W., Berkowitz, A. S., and Keel, B. A.,** Quantitation of LH subunits released by rat anterior pituitary cells in primary culture, *Mol. Cell. Endocrinol.,* 35, 121, 1984.

35. **Keel, B. A., Schanbacher, B. D., and Grotjan, H. E., Jr.,** Ovine luteinizing hormone. II. Effects of castration and steroid administration on the levels of uncombined subunits within the pituitary, *Biol. Reprod.,* 36, 1114, 1987.

36. **Parsons, T. F. and Pierce, J. G.,** Free α-like material from bovine pituitaries. Removal of its o-linked oligosaccharide permits combination with lutropin-β, *J. Biol. Chem.,* 259, 2662, 1984.

37. **Wakabayashi, K.,** Heterogeneity of rat luteinizing hormone revealed by radioimmunoassay and electrofocusing studies, *Endocrinol. Jpn.,* 24, 473, 1977.

38. **Robertson, D. M., Foulds, L. M., and Ellis, S.,** Heterogeneity of rat pituitary gonadotropins on electrofocusing: differences between sexes and after castration, *Endocrinology,* 111, 385, 1982.

39. **Chappel, S. C., Ulloa-Aguirre, A., and Ramaley, J. A.,** Sexual maturation in female rats: time-related changes in the isoelectric focusing pattern of anterior pituitary follicle-stimulating hormone, *Biol. Reprod.,* 28, 196, 1983.

40. **Keel, B. A. and Grotjan, H. E., Jr.,** Characterization or rat lutropin charge microheterogeneity using chromatofocusing, *Anal. Biochem.,* 142, 267, 1984.

41. **Matteri, R. L. and Papkoff, H.,** Characterization of equine luteinizing hormone by chromatofocusing, *Biol. Reprod.,* 36, 261, 1987.

42. **Ulloa-Aguirre, A. and Chappel, S.,** Multiple species of follicle-stimulating hormone exist within the anterior pituitary gland of male golden hamsters, *J. Endocrinol.,* 95, 257, 1982.

43. **Hattori, M. A., Sakamoto, K., and Wakabayashi, K.,** The presence of LH components having different ratios of bioactivity to immunoreactivity in the rat pituitary glands, *Endocrinol. Jpn.,* 30, 289, 1983.

44. **Miller, C., Ulloa-Aguirre, A., Hyland, L., and Chappel, S.,** Pituitary follicle-stimulating hormone heterogeneity:assessment of biological activities of each follicle-stimulating hormone form, *Fertil. Steril.,* 40, 242, 1983.

45. **Peckham, W. D. and Knobil, E.,** Qualitative changes in the pituitary gonadotropins of the male rhesus monkey following castration, *Endocrinology,* 98, 1061, 1976.

46. **Keel, B. A. and Grotjan, H. E., Jr.,** Characterization of rat pituitary luteinizing hormone charge microheterogeneity in male and female rats using chromatofocusing: effects of castration, *Endocrinology,* 117, 354, 1985.

47. **Keel, B. A., Schanbacher, B. D., and Grotjan, H. E., Jr.,** Ovine luteinizing hormone. I. Effects of castration and steroid administration on the charge microheterogeneity of pituitary LH, *Biol. Reprod.,* 36, 1102, 1987.

48. **Keel, B. A. and Grotjan, H. E., Jr.,** Influence of bilateral cryptorchidism on rat pituitary luteinizing hormone charge microheterogeneity, *Biol. Reprod.,* 32, 83, 1985.

49. **Peckham, W. D. and Knobil, E.,** The effects of ovariectomy, estrogen replacement and neuraminidase treatment on the properties of the adenohypophysial glycoprotein hormones on the rhesus monkey, *Endocrinology,* 98, 1054, 1976.

50. **Keel, B. A. and Schanbacher, B. D.,** Charge microheterogeneity of ovine follicle-stimulating hormone in rams and steroid-treated wethers, *Biol. Reprod.,* 37, 386, 1987.

51. **Au, C. L., Robertson, D. M., and de Kretser, D. M.,** In vitro bioassay of inhibin in testes of normal and cryptorchid rats, *Endocrinology,* 112, 239, 1983.

52. **Schanbacher, B. D., Keel, B. A., and Grotjan, H. E., Jr.,** unpublished data, 1989.

Chapter 5

ALTERATIONS IN LEYDIG CELL MORPHOLOGY

Momokazu Gotoh, Koji Miyake, and Hideo Mitsuya

TABLE OF CONTENTS

I. INTRODUCTION

Leydig[1] first described the interstitial cells in the testis, which have since been known as Leydig cells. Bouin and Ancel[2] postulated that these cells were involved in the synthesis of androgenic steroid hormones. Since then, a body of evidence has accumulated, both cytological and biochemical, to confirm their views.[3-8] It is now well established that testosterone is produced from pregnenolone by a series of reactions carried out by enzymes sequestered in the mitochondria and smooth endoplasmic reticulum of Leydig cells.[8,9] It is likewise widely accepted that testosterone synthesized by Leydig cells is essential for maintaining and stimulating normal spermatogenesis.[10]

In cases of cryptorchidism, sterility and subfertility are frequently observed, however, the precise nature of the pathogenesis of the sterility remains unknown. Morphological alterations in the histological components of human and experimental animal cryptorchid testes have been intensively described by numerous investigators, in particular the germ cells in the seminiferous tubules.[11-13] However, only a limited number of reports have appeared on Leydig cell morphology in cryptorchid testes, and some authors described Leydig cells as being not only morphologically, but also functionally, normal in such testes.[14-16] In contrast, evidence suggesting impaired Leydig cell function has recently been reported on human and experimental animal cryptorchid testes, by means of endocrinological, biochemical, and morphological studies.[17-23] In this chapter, morphological alterations in Leydig cells from cryptorchid testis will be reviewed in terms of cellular hypertrophy and hyperplasia, together with cytological changes in each cell structure.

II. DEVELOPMENT AND MORPHOLOGY OF THE NORMAL LEYDIG CELL

It is generally accepted that Leydig cells in the testis derive from mesenchymal cells,[24] which can be transformed into fibroblasts as well as precursor Leydig cells. Ultrastructures of Leydig cells in human fetal testis were precisely described by Niemi and Pelliniemi,[25] Gondos and Hobel,[26] and Holstein.[27] Well-differentiated Leydig cells appear in the interstitium of the human fetal testis at the 8th week. During the period from the 9th to the 12th week, the size of the cell body markedly increases and cell organelles such as Golgi complexes and smooth endoplasmic reticulum develop in the cytoplasm. The development of Leydig cell reaches a maximum between the 12th and the 14th week. After the 14th week, most Leydig cells begin to undergo regressive changes and decline markedly in size and number after the 17th week.

Based on previous light microscopic studies on the development of human Leydig cells after birth,[28-30] it was originally suggested that these cells were not visible before puberty but developed only after puberty. In contrast, however, Hayashi and Harrison[31] claimed that Leydig cells could be visualized in the testis at 1 year of age, but then disappeared, reappearing at around 5 or 6 years of age followed by a continuous increase in size and number until puberty.

There have been a limited number of reports on electron microscopic observations of postnatal Leydig cell development. Hadžieselimović[32] described two basic types of Leydig cells that could be identified in the testis during childhood: precursor and fully developed Leydig cells. According to his observations, both cells are visible in the interstitium throughout childhood. In the development of the Leydig cell, two regressive phases were observed; the first in the 2nd and 3rd year and the second occurs from age 9 to 11. In these regressive periods, mature Leydig cells were nearly absent but precursor cells were observed. After 13 years of age, the Leydig cells increased in size and became further differentiated, and the precursor cells could hardly be detected.

Precursor Leydig cells are similar to the immature fusiform interstitial cell described by

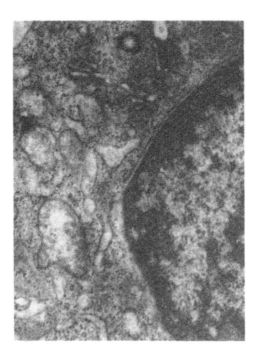

FIGURE 1. Immature precursor cell with scanty cell organelles in the undescended testis of a prepubertal patient. (5-year-old cryptorchid patient, magnification × 19,000.)

Fawcett.[33] These cells have a small cytoplasmic volume containing a small number of mitochondria of cristae type, small and poorly developed Golgi complexes and irregularly shaped nuclei with occasional invaginations, and usually lacking cytoplasmic inclusions such as lipid droplets, pigment granules and Reinke crystalloids (Figure 1). In the cytoplasm, endoplasmic reticulum is not well developed, however, rough endoplasmic reticulum is rather more prominent than smooth endoplasmic reticulum. Glycogen and ribosome granules were dispersed throughout the cytoplasm. The ground cytoplasm has fine filaments lying parallel to each other, which are characteristic of this cell type but disappear in the mature type of Leydig cells (Figure 2).

Ultrastructural properties of mature Leydig cells have been recorded by Fawcett,[33] Yamada,[5] and de Kretser.[6] Leydig cells are usually observed in groups, even though isolated cells are likewise encountered. Typical mature Leydig cells in the normal human testis show a large cytoplasm embedding a round nucleus, which is usually located excentrically (Figure 3). The cells are generally polygonal or round in shape, but occasionally extend slender or irregular processes. The nucleus contains relatively dispersed heterochromatin particles and usually one prominent nucleolus. A small amount of condensed heterochromatin is recognized along the inner leaflet of the nuclear envelope (Figure 4). The cytoplasm contains mitochondria, endoplasmic reticulum, Golgi complexes, lipid droplets, glycogen particles, pigment granules, and Reinke crystalloids (Figure 5). The most prominent feature of Leydig cells is the presence of extensively developed smooth endoplasmic reticulum throughout the entire cytoplasm (Figure 4). The reticulum is vesicular or tubular in appearance and relatively uniform in diameter. The degree of development of the smooth endoplasmic reticulum varies to some extent from cell to cell in the same specimen. It is probable that these variations reflect differences in their physiological state with respect to the production or storage of secretory products. In the majority of cells, however, the smooth endoplasmic reticulum is

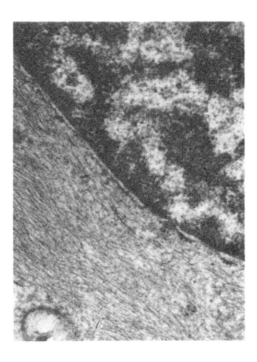

FIGURE 2.   The cytoplasm of an immature precursor cell exhibiting fine fibrils. (5-year-old cryptorchid patient, magnification × 30,000.)

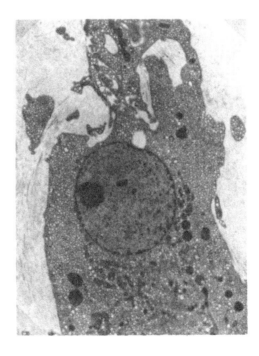

FIGURE 3.   A Leydig cell from a normal testis of a 33-year-old fertile man. It has a round nucleus and wide cytoplasm containing abundant cell organelles. (Magnification × 3600.)

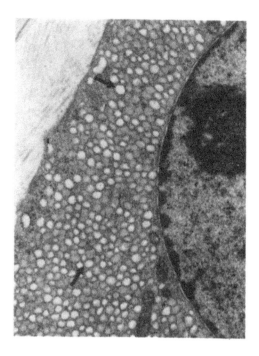

FIGURE 4. A portion of a Leydig cell from a normal testis of a 33-year-old fertile man. The elements of smooth endoplasmic reticulum (arrows) are extensively developed. (Magnification × 13,000.)

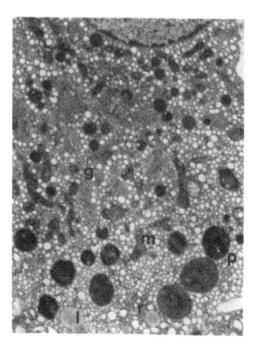

FIGURE 5. A portion of a Leydig cell from a normal testis of a 25-year-old fertile man. A variety of organelles are well developed in the cytoplasm: Golgi complex (g), lipid droplet (l), lipochrome pigment granule (p), mitochondria (m), and ribosome granule (r). (27-year-old normal adult, magnification × 6000.)

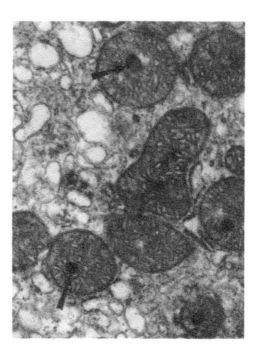

FIGURE 6.   Mitochondria in the cytoplasm of a normal
Leydig cell. Some of them contain electron-dense gran-
ules(arrows). (26 year-old normal adult, magnification ×
24,000.)

so well developed and so compactly packed that the space between the reticulum is greatly
reduced. The reticulum appears empty or less opaque than the surrounding cytoplasmic
matrix. The rough endoplasmic reticulum is tubular in feature and occurs infrequently in
small number. Mitochondria are usually recognized in the cytoplasm and are occasionally
found in abundance. They vary in size and shape; they are usually oval or spherical, whereas
elongated or tubular forms are at times observed. The majority appear in section to be simple
plications of the inner membrane, however they occasionally form loops or more complicated
arrangements. At times they contain one or more electron-dense bodies in their matrix (Figure
6). Golgi complexes are well developed in a juxtanuclear area, consisting of curved parallel
arrays of layered, flattened sacs and vesicles (Figure 5). A number of aggregations of
moderately osmiophilic material, which are referred to as lipid droplets, are noted (Figure
5). The majority of these lipid droplets are encapsulated within expanded smooth-surfaced
vesicles. Occasionally, their contents are partly extracted and exhibit less-electron opacities.
They vary in size and location. Deposits of intensely osmiophilic lipochrome pigments,
generally membrane bounded, are found scattered throughout the cytoplasm (Figure 5). In
addition to these deposits, a number of small granules of ribosome and glycogen are seen
scattered throughout the cytoplasmic matrix. Crystalloids of Reinke[34] may be found irregularly scattered in the cytoplasm. The location, number, and size, as well as configuration,
of the crystalloids vary greatly. At high magnification, precisely periodic structures are
visible in the crystalloids (Figure 7). Such crystalloids are believed to occur after puberty
in the normal development of human testis.

III. LEYDIG CELL HYPERPLASIA AND HYPERTROPHY IN THE CRYPTORCHID TESTIS

Leydig cell hyperplasia has been reported to occur under a variety of pathological conditions in the testes such as after X-ray irradiation,[35] Klinefelter's syndrome,[36] and varico-

FIGURE 7. Reinke crystalloid, showing a regular crystalline structure of hexagonal, honeycomb patterns. (33-year-old normal adult, magnification × 26,000.)

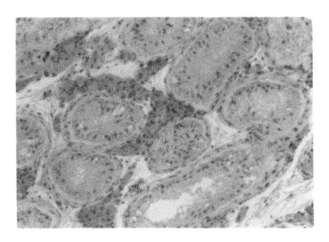

FIGURE 8. The undescended testis of a postpubertal cryptorchid patient (32 years old).

cele,[37] and it has often been found in association with distorted spermatogenesis. In cryptorchidism, Leydig cell hyperplasia has likewise been substantiated by light microscopy in undescended testes of experimental animals[38] and adult cryptorchid patients[39] (Figure 8), even though other workers[14-16] have suggested that Leydig cells were normal in such testes. In most of these studies, however, Leydig cell hyperplasia was evaluated on the basis of rough and subjective data obtained by microscopic observation on biopsied specimens. In testes with impaired spermatogenesis of any etiologies, decrease in diameter of the seminiferous tubules is frequently recognized. On subjective observation of histologic section with light microscopy, Leydig cell hyperplasia may be taken to be an artifact due to the decrease in size of the seminiferous tubules. Weiss et al.[40] recorded a simple method for the quantitative evaluation of Leydig cell number. They have revealed a significant correlation among three indices of Leydig cell number: (1) Leydig cells per seminiferous tubule, (2) Leydig cells per cluster, and (3) Leydig cell clusters per seminiferous tubule. They suggested that the best index for practical clinical use could be the ratio of Leydig cell clusters per seminiferous tubule in favor of its simplicity. This method was first employed for the quantitative evaluation of Leydig cell number in cryptorchid testes by Gotoh et al.[41] In light microscopy, the total number of seminiferous tubules, Leydig cells, Leydig cell clusters, and Sertoli cells were counted in all the histologic sections of biopsied testicular specimens from human cryptorchid patients. In consequence, indices of Leydig cells per seminiferous tubule, Leydig cell clusters per seminiferous tubule, Leydig cells per cluster, and Leydig cell-Sertoli cell ratio were determined. Leydig cells per seminiferous tubule was calculated by dividing the total number of Leydig cells counted in the entire histologic sections by the total number of seminiferous tubules. Leydig cell clusters per seminiferous tubule was determined by dividing the number of Leydig cell clusters by the total number of seminiferous tubules. Leydig cells per cluster was obtained by dividing the total number of Leydig cells in the clusters by the number of clusters counted in the entire sections. The Leydig-Sertoli cell ratio was estimated by dividing the total number of Leydig cells counted in the entire histologic sections by the total number of Sertoli cells in seminiferous tubules. In that study, tissue specimens were obtained from ten undescended testes and four contralateral scrotal testes of postpubertal cryptorchid patients and from six normal testes of fertile adults. A significant correlation was substantiated among these indices (Figure 9). When the indices of the undescended and contralateral scrotal testes of the cryptorchid patients were compared with those of normal individuals, all the indices were significantly higher in both undescended and descended scrotal testes of the patients than in those of the normal controls (Figure 10). Furthermore, all the indices of Leydig cell number tended to be higher in the contralateral scrotal testes than in the undescended ones (Figure 10). According to previous subjective observations[38,39] and these quantitative data,[41] it is certain that Leydig cell hyperplasia is present in the undescended testes of postpubertal cryptorchid patients, and it is most interesting that this is also the case with the contralateral scrotal testes.

Leydig cell hypertrophy has been described in a variety of conditions. Rich[42] observed hypertrophy of Leydig cells in the testes of rats with disturbed spermatogenesis induced by experimental means such as fetal irradiation, vitamin A deficiency, and hydroxyurea treatment. Clegg[43] interpreted Leydig cell hyperplasia and hypertrophy as reflecting compensatory changes in the contralateral scrotal testis of experimental unilateral cryptorchidism in rats. In surgically induced cryptorchid testes of rats, Kerr[44] recorded Leydig cell hypertrophy, as revealed by a doubling of cell and nuclear volume and by ultrastructural morphometry. On the other hand, other investigators have noted in human cryptorchid testes that most Leydig cells were atrophic and small in size with various regressive changes in cell organelles on ultrastructural observation.[32,45] Unlike Leydig cell hyperplasia, confirmative objective data have not been obtained yet to verify the presence of Leydig cell hypertrophy in cryptorchid human testes.

IV. ULTRASTRUCTURAL ALTERATIONS OF LEYDIG CELL IN THE CRYPTORCHID TESTIS

In light microscopy, a number of authors were able to identify changes in number of Leydig cells only after puberty.[29,39,46] Cytologic observation with electron microscopy was needed to clarify the qualitative and functional alterations in Leydig cells. Few reports are available on ultrastructural alterations in Leydig cells from human and even experimental

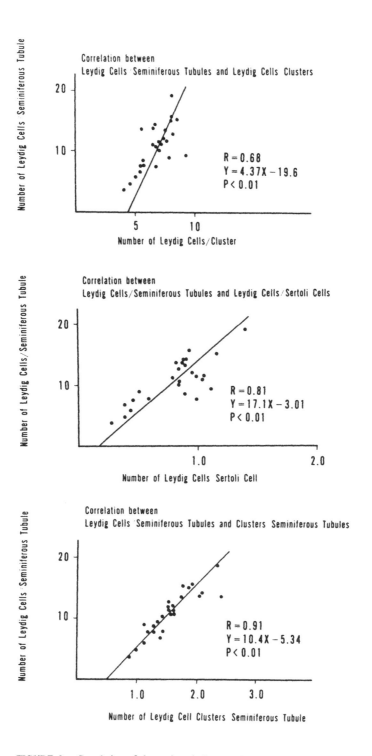

FIGURE 9. Correlation of the various indices to the mean number of Leydig cells per seminiferous tubule.

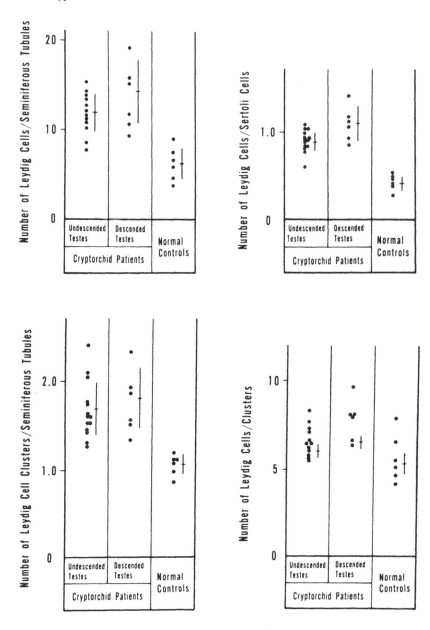

FIGURE 10.   Comparison of each index in cryptorchid patients and normal controls.

animal cryptorchid testes. Numanoglu[11] revealed a lack of Leydig cell development beginning at 5 years of age and continuing to a maximum of 13 to 15 years of age, substantiated by fewer and less dense mitochondria and less developed smooth endoplasmic reticulum in the cytoplasm. Hadžiselimovic[32] investigated Leydig cell morphology in cryptorchid boys aged 1 to 15 years, comparing it with that of normal control Leydig cells from the same age group. He found Leydig cells lying singly in the interstitium in cryptorchid testes of 1-year-old patients. Their cytoplasm was much thinner than in normal control Leydig cells from the same age group. Occasionally, Leydig cells were atrophic or degenerating, containing an irregular-shaped nucleus with numerous invaginations. The cytoplasm of these atrophic Leydig cells was provided with fewer uncharacteristic cell organelles, mitochondria, and lipid droplets. Smooth endoplasmic reticulum was very scarce, and large empty vacuoles

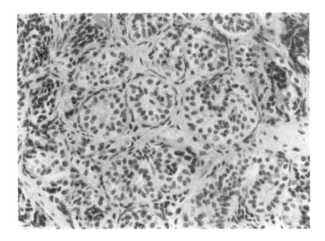

FIGURE 11. The undescended testis of a prepubertal cryptorchid patient (5 years old).

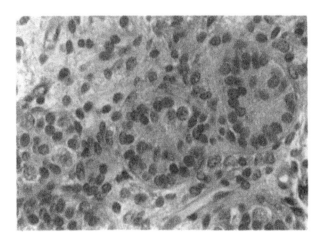

FIGURE 12. The undescended testis of a 5-year-old cryptorchid patient, treated preoperatively by 20,000 IU of hCG.

were commonly encountered in the cytoplasm of these cells. It was likewise observed that from the 1st year until puberty, mature type Leydig cells were exceedingly rare in the interstitium, and, in puberty, Leydig cell development was found to be retarded.

Our own observations on Leydig cells were performed on cryptorchid patients aged 3 to 37 years, and focused on the structural alterations in precursor and mature Leydig cells. In prepubertal patients, Leydig cells were usually of the immature precursor type, with fusiform-shaped cytoplasm containing prominent cytoplasmic fine filaments and few organelles; mature Leydig cells were seldom detected (Figure 11). However, in the cryptorchid testis of the patients (5 to 7 years old) who had received a human chorionic gonadotropin (hCG) injection preoperatively, mature type Leydig cells could be identified both light (Figure 12) and electron (Figure 13) microscopically. During pubertal periods, although mature Leydig cells were occasionally detected, immature cells were still prominent, substantiating the previous findings by Hadžiselimovič, i.e., retarded development of Leydig cells in puberty. In the testes of postpubertal patients, most Leydig cells had usually developed into mature type cells. However, such mature Leydig cells as appeared in the testes of pubertal and

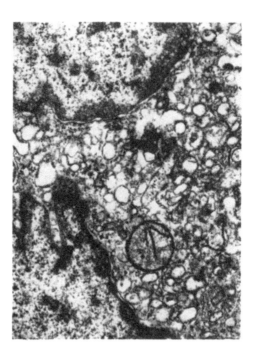

FIGURE 13.   A portion of a Leydig cell from the undescended testis of a 5-year-old cryptorchid patient, treated
preoperatively by hCG. The cytoplasm is provided with
abundant elements of smooth endoplasmic reticulum.
(Magnification × 22,000.)

postpubertal patients, frequently underwent morphological changes as follows: the cytoplasm
tended to be thin and the nuclear envelope often revealed an undulated contour and at times
deep invaginations (Figure 14). The most prominent alteration visualized in the cytoplasm
was a decline in number and an unevenness in size of the smooth endoplasmic reticulum
(Figures 15 and 16). Vesicular elements of reticulum were distended occasionally and showed
irregular contours. With the decline of smooth endoplasmic reticulum, the space between
the reticulum was enlarged. Leydig cells containing markedly developed rough endoplasmic
reticulum were rarely detected, probably reflecting the immaturity of the cells. In addition,
empty vacuoles were occasionally found in the cytoplasm. Mitochondria were variable in
size, and oval, spherical, or tubular in shape. They contained occasional intramitochondrial
bodies, even though the number of mitochondria in the cytoplasm tended to be low (Figure
16). Their morphological features revealed no prominent differences from those of normal
controls. Golgi complex was, on the whole, poorly developed, and occupied merely a smaller
juxtanuclear region in the cytoplasm (Figure 15). Lipid droplets in the cytoplasm were
relatively few, and smaller in size. On the other hand, tiny highly osmiophilic granules,
which were referred to as ribosome or glycogen granules, were recognized in increased
numbers diffused or aggregated in the spaces between the endoplasmic reticulum. Some
cells contained cytoplasmic fine filaments, which could not be detected in normal mature
cells. The crystalloids of Reinke were visualized in the undescended testis after 12 years of
age. In location, number, size, and ultrastructural features of the crystalloids, no prominent
difference from normal controls could be detected. Another particular feature of Leydig cells
in the cryptorchid testis was the presence of cytoplasmic inclusion bodies noted only in the
postpubertal patients. These inclusion bodies had fascicular features, and exhibited two
different modes of distribution in the cytoplasm: some of them appeared as disseminated
groups of few subunits (Figures 16 and 17), but scattered preferentially in the juxtanuclear

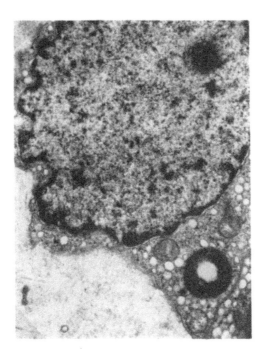

FIGURE 14. A portion of a Leydig cell from the undescended testis of a 19-year-old cryptorchid patient. The nuclear envelope is irregular in shape with occasional invaginations, and the cytoplasm possesses less smooth endoplasmic reticulum. (Magnification × 11,000.)

sites; whereas others were seen as large aggregates of subunits which were islet-like in appearance (Figure 18). The subunits forming the inclusion bodies exhibited fasciculate structures composed of several parallel arrays of electron-dense substances (Figure 19). In cross sections, these structures were found to be arranged in loop- or ring-shaped configurations (Figure 20). In this study, the inclusion bodies mentioned were likewise found in Leydig cells of both the contralateral descended testes of the patients and the testes of normal controls. However, they appeared with greater frequency in the undescended testes. Furthermore, the inclusion bodies were prominent in Leydig cells that underwent the morphological alterations mentioned above. Yamada[5] reported the presence of inclusion bodies similar to those described above in Leydig cells from normal testes and postulated that they represent a possible precursor of the Reinke crystalloid. These crystalloids have likewise been observed in Leydig cells from adult infertile patients[47] and patients with Klinefelter's syndrome.[48] Since the inclusion bodies were identified predominantly in Leydig cells undergoing regressive changes, and the ultrastructure of these inclusions was apparently different from that of Reinke crystalloids, these structures are more likely related to some pathological change of Leydig cells rather than representing a precursor of Reinke crystalloids. In testes from patients with Klinefelter's syndrome, Smith et al.[48] noticed that these inclusion bodies disappeared following androgen treatment, suggesting a possible relationship between the inclusion bodies and the metabolism of male sex hormones.

It has often been reported that sterility and subfertility are frequent not only in bilateral cryptorchids but also in unilateral cryptorchid patients. A number of investigators have noted pathological changes in the descended scrotal testis of unilateral cryptorchid patients, particularly pronounced in germ cells. Shirai et al.,[49] using experimentally cryptorchid dogs, noted histologically extensive degenerative changes in germ cells and hence suppressed

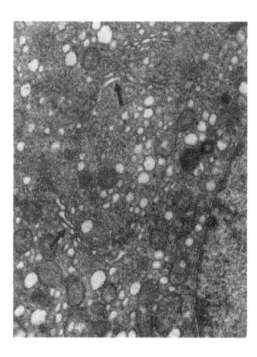

FIGURE 15.   A portion of a Leydig cell from the undescended testis of a 19-year-old patient. Golgi complex
(arrows) is poorly developed and a depletion in the extent
of smooth endoplasmic reticulum is observed. (Magnification × 14,000.)

spermatogenesis both in cryptorchid and contralateral scrotal testes. On Leydig cells in
contralateral scrotal testis of unilateral cryptorchids, however, there has been no data to
reveal particular histological or cytological abnormalities, except the Leydig cell hyperplasia
described previously.[41]

IV. RELATIONSHIP BETWEEN LEYDIG CELL MORPHOLOGY AND FUNCTION IN THE CRYPTORCHID TESTIS

Extensively developed smooth endoplasmic reticulum in the cytoplasm, uniformly noted
in steroid hormone-producing cells, is the most characteristic finding of mature Leydig cells.
Leydig cells are further characterized by the presence of prominent mitochondria and abundant lipid droplets, which are also common features among cells which produce steroid
hormone. Mitochondria are present in abundance and relatively large in size, with occasional
intramitochondrial granules. These cell organelles are believed to play prominent roles in
testosterone synthesis of Leydig cells.[8,9] The lipid droplets are reported to contain esterified
cholesterol which serves as a source of cholesterol in testosterone synthesis.[50] Mitochondria
contain the enzyme complex responsible for the conversion of cholesterol to pregnenolone.[50]
The smooth endoplasmic reticulum contains a series of enzymes which convert pregnenolone
to testosterone.[51,52] Relationships of Leydig cell number, volume, or ultrastructure with
testicular steroidogenic activity have been investigated by numerous authors under a variety
of experimental conditions.[53-59] It has been generally concluded that Leydig cell number
and/or volume correlate with testosterone concentration in peripheral blood and in the testis,
and that there are striking changes in the smooth endoplasmic reticulum and lipid droplets
accompanying the changes in testicular steroidogenic activity. Zirkin et al.[60] demonstrated

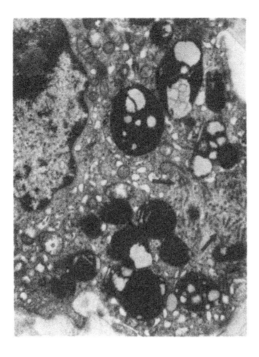

FIGURE 16. A degenerating Leydig cell from the undescended testis of a 30-year-old cryptorchid patient. It
has marked regressive changes. Cytoplasmic inclusion
bodies (arrows) are detected. (Magnification × 9600.)

a linear positive correlation between testosterone secretion and the amount of smooth endoplasmic reticulum in Leydig cells from five animal species. Based on these findings, there
is no doubt that a significant association exists between Leydig cell morphology and steroidogenic function.

Despite numerous investigations, the precise etiology of undescendence of the testis in
cryptorchidism remains unanswered. Originally, congenital anatomical anomalies of gubernaculum, inguinal canal, vas deferens, spermatic vessels, and/or cremaster muscle were
postulated as being responsible for undescendence of the testis. On the other hand, since
Shapiro[61] first reported that hCG administration could lead to descendence of cryptorchid
testes in young children, it has been hypothesized that undescendence of the testis might be
due to deficient LH stimulation of Leydig cells during the fetal period. Raynaud[62] and Jean[63]
induced uni- or bilateral cryptorchidism in male mice following estrogen administration to
gravid mice. Using the same technique, Hadžiselimovič and Girard[64] succeeded in inducing
cryptorchid mice and made light and electron microscopic study of Leydig cells. They could
detect atrophic and degenerated Leydig cells in the undescended testis of the estrogen-treated
newborn mice, but not in the testis of normal controls. These atrophic changes in Leydig
cells of newborn mice could nearly be eliminated by simultaneous administration of both
hCG and estrogen to their mothers. Further, they noted that the atrophic Leydig cells found
in the estrogen-treated mice were extremely similar to those observed in cryptorchid testis
in 1-year-old patients. These experimental data support the hypothesis that undescendence
of the testis might be the result of deficient Leydig cell function during the fetal period.

Mature Leydig cells are known to differentiate from immature precursor cells under the
influence of LH stimulation.[29,65,66] The aforementioned morphological changes in mature
Leydig cells in the human from postnatal to pubertal periods correlate to changes in sex
hormone metabolism. Charny[67] and Hadžiselimovič[32] detected a number of mature Leydig

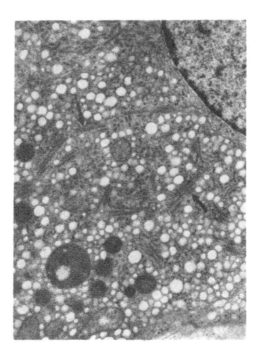

FIGURE 17.   A portion of a Leydig cell from the undescended testis of a 26-year-old patient. Cytoplasmic
inclusion bodies (arrows) consisting of groups of a few
subunits are scattered in the cytoplasm. The elements of
smooth endoplasmic reticulum are fewer and more irregular in size than in the Leydig cells in normal testes.
(Magnification × 25,000.)

cells during the neonatal period and at 1 year of age. Forest[68] revealed an increase in plasma
testosterone level during the initial 3 months after birth. The elevated plasma testosterone
level beginning at puberty is likewise consistent with the morphological findings that well-
developed, mature Leydig cells rapidly increase in number during the pubertal period.

Leydig cell function was initially believed to be normal in cryptorchid patients in view
of the normal development of secondary sex characteristics in puberty. Recently, however,
hormonal abnormalities have been described by several investigators. In rats surgically made
cryptorchid, a diminution in amount of extractable androgen was reported in the undescended
testes.[69] In dogs, Eiknes[70] noted a lower concentration of testosterone in venous blood from
the undescended testis than in that from the contralateral scrotal testis. The activities of
enzymes directly involved in steroidogenesis declined in Leydig cells of undescended testes
of rats.[23] In the human, Raboch[18] revealed a diminution in plasma testosterone levels in
postpubertal bilateral cryptorchid patients. Kodaira,[20] employing his specific technique,
noticed that androgen production was suppressed in the undescended testis of human cryptorchid patients after 5 years of age, as compared with the testes of normal individuals of
the same age. Gendrel[71] showed that in both bi- and unilateral cryptorchids the postnatal
testosterone rise during the initial 3 months was significantly lower than that in normal
controls. Only a small number of reports have been presented on alterations in pituitary
function of cryptorchid patients. Job[19] described impaired LH secretion in response to LH-
RH in prepubertal cryptorchid patients, suggesting a possible decreased pituitary reserve of
LH. Delayed plasma testosterone elevation during puberty[21,22] and elevated plasma LH level
after puberty[21,72,73] have also been reported in human cryptorchids.

The previous section described the marked decline in the mature Leydig cell population

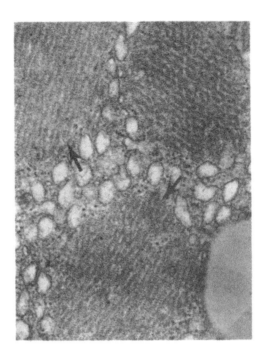

FIGURE 18. A portion of the cytoplasm of a Leydig cell from the undescended testis of a 30-year-old cryptorchid patient. Cytoplasmic inclusion bodies (arrows) consisting of large aggregates of subunits are islet-like in appearance. (Magnification × 37,000.)

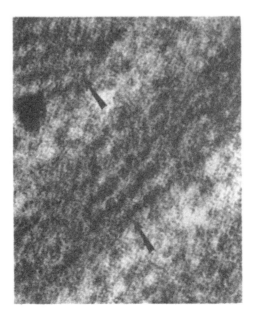

FIGURE 19. High power view of a longitudinal section through the subunits forming cytoplasmic inclusion bodies. Each subunit (arrows) contains several parallel arrays of electron dense structures consisting of aggregations of curved or coiled canaliculi embedded in opaque granules. (Magnification × 190,000.)

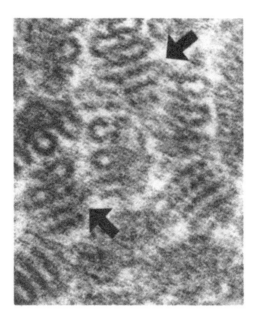

FIGURE 20.　High power view of cross-section through the subunits forming cytoplasmic inclusion bodies. In each subunit (arrows), groups of arrays are arranged in loop- or ring-shaped configurations. (Magnification × 220,000.)

in cryptorchid testes from the neonatal to pubertal periods, and the cytological alterations in mature Leydig cells, especially in the cytoplasmic components closely related to testosterone synthesis. These findings are believed to reflect decreased testosterone synthesis in Leydig cells in undescended testis during these periods. Kodaira[74] and Gotoh et al.[45] noted that, following administration of hCG, mature Leydig cells increased in number in the undescended testis of prepubertal patients. Together with Job's[19] report which revealed a diminished pituitary LH reserve in prepubertal patients, these data might imply that the poor development of mature Leydig cells in the prepubertal cryptorchid testis is due to deficient LH stimulation.

It was shown that after puberty mature Leydig cells increased in number, but that the majority of these cells underwent various degress of regressive changes which were especially pronounced in smooth endoplasmic reticulum, Golgi complexes, mitochondria, and lipid droplets. These data strongly suggest that, despite the increased number of Leydig cells, total Leydig cell function declines in the postpubertal cryptorchid testis. These morphological findings are further substantiated by the decline in testosterone synthesis in such testes. Since Leydig cells in the contralateral scrotal testis usually remained morphologically intact, certain local factors, such as high temperature must be additionally responsible for the regressive changes noted in mature Leydig cells of the postpubertal cryptorchid testis.

The exact mechanism underlying Leydig cell hyperplasia remains unknown. Inaba et al.[75] revealed Leydig cell hyperplasia in undescended testes and increased plasma LH levels in rats with experimentally produced cryptorchidism. These authors further reported that such phenomena were eliminated in hypophysectomized rats. In human, they noted plasma LH elevation after puberty in cryptorchids. It can be hypothesized that Leydig cell hyperplasia observed in the postpubertal cryptorchid testis, and probably also in the contralateral scrotal testis, might represent a compensatory change induced by LH elevation in response to the primary Leydig cell dysfunction in the cryptorchid testis.

V. CONCLUSION

In this chapter, morphological alterations of Leydig cells in the cryptorchid testis have been described for the fetal, prepubertal, pubertal, and postpubertal periods. These data are consistent with the hormonal abnormalities recognized in such patients and suggest a functional impairment of Leydig cell in terms of testosterone production. Sufficient intratesticular concentration of testosterone, namely normal Leydig cell function, is responsible for the normal development and maintenance of other testicular components such as germ cells, Sertoli cells, and the seminiferous tubular wall. Active spermatogenesis is likewise regulated by testosterone. The Leydig cell dysfunction suggested in cryptorchid testes therefore, could be closely correlated with the deficient spermatogenesis in this disorder. Since the exact nature of pathogenesis of sterility in cryptorchidism is not fully understood, the interrelationships between Leydig cell dysfunction and other testicular components is an important key subject worthy of further critical investigation.

REFERENCES

1. **Leydig, F.,** Zur Anatomie der menschlichen Geschlechtsorgane und Analdrüsen der Säugetiere, *Z. Wiss. Zool.,* 2, 1, 1850.
2. **Bouin, P. and Ancel, P.,** Recherches sur le cellules interstitielles du testicles chez les mammiferes, *Arch. Zool. Exp. Gen.,* 1, 437, 1903.
3. **Ito, T. and Oinuma, S.,** Cytologische Untersuchungen uber die Hodenzwischenzellen des Menschen mit besonderer Berucksichtigung auf die Bedeutung von Lipoid und Pigment, *Fol. Anat. Jpn.,* 18, 497, 1939.
4. **Fawcett, D. W. and Burgos, M. H.,** Studies on the fine structure of mammalian testes. II. The human interstitial tissue, *Am. J. Anat.,* 107, 245, 1960.
5. **Yamada, E.,** Some observations on the fine structure of the interstitial cell in the human testis as revealed by electron microscopy, *Gumma Symp. Endocrinol.,* 2, 1, 1965.
6. **de Kretser, D. M.,** The fine structure of the testicular interstitial cells in men of normal androgenic status, *Z. Zellforsch.,* 80, 594, 1967.
7. **Shikita, M. and Tamaoki, B.,** Testosterone formation by subcellular particles of rat testis, *Endocrinology,* 76, 563, 1965.
8. **Tamaoki, B. and Shikita, M.,** Biosynthesis of steroids in testicular tissue in vitro, in *Steroid Dynamics,* Pincus, G., Makao, T., and Tart, J. F., Eds., Academic Press, New York, 1966, 493.
9. **Hall, P. F.,** Testicular hormones synthesis and control, in *Endocrinology,* Vol. 3, DeGroot, L. J., Cahill, G. F., Jr., and Odell, W. D., Eds., Grune & Stratton, New York, 1979, 1511.
10. **Steinberger, E.,** Hormonal control of mammalian spermatogenesis, Physiol. Rev., 51, 1, 1971.
11. **Numanoglu, I., Köktürk, I., and Mutaf, O.,** Light and electron microscopic examinations of undescended testicles, *J. Pediatr. Sugr.,* 4, 614, 1969.
12. **Leeson, C. R.,** An electron microscopic study of cryptorchid and scrotal human testes with special reference to pubertal maturation, *Invest. Urol.,* 3, 498, 1966.
13. **Plöen, L.,** An electron microscopic study of the delayed effects on rabbit spermatogenesis following experimental cryptorchidism for twenty-four hours, *Virchows Arch. B,* 14, 159, 1973.
14. **Daniel, D. F.,** *Abnormal Sexual Development,* W.B. Saunders, Philadelphis, 1969, 146.
15. **Mancini, R. E., Rosemberg, E., and Cullen, M,** Cryptorchid and scrotal human testes. I. Cytological, cyotchemical and quantitative studies, *J. Clin. Endocrinol.,* 25, 927, 1964.
16. **Williams, R. H.,** *Textbook of Endocrinology,* 5th ed., W.B. Saunders, Philadelphia, 1974, 357.
17. **Engberg, H.,** Investigation of the endocrine function of the testicle in cryptorchidism, *Proc. R. Soc. Med.,* 42, 652, 1969.
18. **Raboch, J. and Starka, L.,** Plasmatic testosterone in bilateral cryptorchids in adult age, *Andrologie,* 4, 107, 1972.
19. **Job, C., Garnier, P. E., and Chaussain, J. E.,** Effect of synthetic luteinizing hormone-releasing hormone on the release of gonadotrophins in hypophysogonadal disorders of children and adolescents. IV. Undescended testis, *J. Pediatr.,* 84, 371, 1974.
20. **Kodaira, T.,** Endocrinological studies on cryptorchidism, Part 1, Reference of androgen biosynthesis of testes, especially in human cryptorchidism, *Jpn. J. Urol.,* 67, 795, 1976.

21. **Waaler, D. E.,** Endocrinological studies in undescended testis, *Acta Pediatr. Scand.,* 65, 559, 1976.
22. **Okuyama, A., Itatani, H., Mizutani, S., Sonoda, T., Aono, T., and Matsumoto, K.,** Pituitary and gonadal function in prepubertal and pubertal cryptorchidism, *Acta Endocrinol.,* 95, 553, 1980.
23. **Kormano, M., Härkönen, M., and Kontinen, E.,** Effect of experimental cryptorchidism on histochemically demonstrable dehydrogenases of the rat testis, *Endocrinology,* 74, 44, 1964.
24. **Hooker, W. Ch.,** The intertubular tissue of the testis, in *The Testis,* Vol. 1, Johnson, A. D., Gomes, W. R. and Vandemark, N. L., Eds., Academic Press, New York, 1970, 488.
25. **Niemi, M. and Pelliniemi, L.,** Fine structure of the human fetal testis. I. The interstitial tissue, *Z. Zellforsch.,* 99, 507, 1969.
26. **Gondos, B. and Hobel, C. J.,** Ultrastructure of germ cell development in the human fetal testis, *Z. Zellforsch.,* 119, 1, 1971.
27. **Holstein, A. F., Wartenbel, H., and Vossmeyer, J.,** Zur Cytologie der pranatalen Gonadenentwicklung beim Menschen, *Z. Anat. Entwickl. Gesch.,* 135, 43, 1971.
28. **Albert, A., Underdahl, L. O., Greene, L. F., and Lorenz, N.,** Male hypogonadism. I. The normal testis, *Mayo Clin. Proc.,* 28, 409, 1953.
29. **Sniffen, R. C.,** The normal testis, *Arch. Pathol.,* 50, 259, 1950.
30. **Mancini, R. E., Vilar, O., Lavieri, J. C., Andrada, J. A., and Heinrich, J. J.,** Development of Leydig cells in the normal human testis. Cytological, cytochemical and quantitative studies, *Am. J. Anat.,* 112, 203, 1963.
31. **Hayashi, H. and Harrison, R. G.,** The development of the interstitial tissue of the human testis, *Fertil. Steril.,* 22, 351, 1971.
32. **Hadžiselimovič, F.,** Cryptorchidism; ultrastructure of normal and cryptorchid testis development, *Adv. Anat. Embryol. Cell. Biol.,* 53, 1, 1977.
33. **Fawcett, D. W. and Burgos, M. H.,** Studies on the fine structure of mammalian testes. II. The human interstitial tissue, *Am. J. Anat.,* 107, 245, 1963.
34. **Reinke, Fr.,** Beiträge zur Histologie des Menschen. I. Uber Krystalloidbildungen in den interstitiellen Zellen des menschlichen Hodens, *Arch. Microscop. Anat.,* 47, 34, 1896.
35. **Blundon, K. E., Russi, S., and Bunts, R. C.,** Interstitial cell hyperplasia or adenoma, *J. Urol.,* 70, 759, 1953.
36. **Klinefelter, H. F., Jr., Reifenstein, E. C., Jr., and Albright, F. J.,** Syndrome characterized by gynecomastia, aspermatogenesis without A-Leydigism and increased excretion of follicle-stimulating hormone, *Clin. Endocrinol.,* 2, 615, 1942.
37. **Dubin, L. and Hotchkiss, R. S.,** Testis biopsy in subfertile men with varicocele, *Fertil. Steril.,* 20, 50, 1969.
38. **Leeson, T. S. and Leeson, C. R.,** Experimental cryptorchidism in the rat; a light and electron microscopic study, *Invest. Urol.,* 8, 124, 1970.
39. **Sohval, A. R.,** Histopathology of cryptorchidism, a study based upon the comparative histology of retained and scrotal testis from birth to maturity, *Am. J. Med.,* 16, 346, 1954.
40. **Weiss, D. B., Rodriguez-Rigau, L., Smith, K. D., Chowdhury, A., and Steinberger, E.,** Quantification of Leydig cells in testicular biopsies of oligospermic men with varicocele, *Fertil. Steril.,* 30, 305, 1978.
41. **Gotoh, M., Miyake, K., and Mitsuya, H.,** Leydig cell hyperplasia in cryptorchid patients; quantitative evaluation of Leydig cells in undescended and contralateral scrotal testes, *Urol. Res.,* 12, 159, 1984.
42. **Rich, K. A., Kerr, J. B., and de Kretser, D. M.,** Evidence for Leydig cell dysfunction in rats with seminiferous tubule damage, *Mol. Cell. Endocrinol.,* 13, 123, 1979.
43. **Clegg, E. J.,** Studies on artificial cryptorchidism; compensatory changes in the scrotal testes of unilateral cryptorchid rats, *J. Endocrinol.,* 33, 259, 1965.
44. **Kerr, J. B., Rich, K. A., and de Kretser, D. M.,** Alterations of the fine structure and androgen secretion of the interstitial cells in the experimentall cryptorchid rat testis, *Biol. Reprod.,* 20, 409, 1979.
45. **Gotoh, M., Miyake, K., and Mitsuya, H.,** A study on cryptorchidism. I. Light and electron microscopic study of Leydig cells in the testes of cryptorchid patients, *Acta Urol. Jpn.,* 30, 327, 1984.
46. **de la Balze, F. A., Mancini, R. E., Arrillaga, F., Andrada, J. A., Vilar, O., Gurtmann, A. I., and Davidson, O. W.,** Histologic study of the undescended human testis during puberty, *J. Clin. Endocrinol.,* 20, 286, 1960.
47. **Hatakeyama, S.,** A study on the interstitial cells of the human testis, especially on their fine structural pathology, *Acta Pathol. Jpn.,* 15, 155, 1965.
48. **Smith, B. D., Leeson, C. R., and Bunge, R. C.,** Microscopic appearance of the testis in Klinefelter's syndrome before and after suppression of gonadotrophin production with testosterone, *Invest. Urol.,* 5, 58, 1967.
49. **Shirai, M., Matsukita, S., Kagayama, M., Ichijo, S., and Taguchi, M.,** Histological changes of the scrotal testis in unilateral cryptorchidism, *Tohoku J. Exp. Med.,* 90, 363, 1966.
50. **Christensen, A. K.,** Leydig cells, in *Handbook of Physiology and Endocrinology,* Vol. 5, Greep, R. O. and Astwood, E. B., Eds., American Physiological Society, Washington, D.C., 1975, 57.

51. **Ewing, L. L. and Brown, B. L.,** Testicular steroidogenesis, in *The Testis,* Vol. 4, Johnson, A. D. and Gomes, W. R., Eds., Academic Press, New York, 1977, 239.

52. **Ewing, L. L., Davis, J. C., and Zirkin, B. R.,** Regulation of testicular function: a spacial and temporal view, in *Reproductive Physiology III,* Vol. 22, Greep, R. O., Ed., International Review of Physiology, University Park Press, Baltimore, 1980, 41.

53. **Christensen, A. K. and Peacock, K. C.,** Increase in Leydig cell number in testes of adult rats treated chronically with an excess of human chorionic gonadotrophin, *Biol. Reprod.,* 22, 383, 1980.

54. **Dym, M. and Raj, H. G. M.,** Response of adult rat Sertoli cells and Leydig cells to depletion of luteinizing hormone and testosterone, *Biol. Reprod.,* 17, 676, 1977.

55. **Gondos, B., Rao, A., and Ramachandran, J.,** Effects of antiserum to luteinizing hormone on the structure and function of rat Leydig cells. *J. Endocrinol.,* 87, 265, 1980.

56. **Nussdorfer, G. G., Robba, C., Mazzocchi, G., and Rebuffat, P.,** Effects of human chorionic gonadotropins on the interstitial cells of the rat testis; a morphometric and radioimmunological study, *Int. J. Androl.,* 3, 319, 1980.

57. **Knorr, D. W., Vanka-Pertula, T., and Lipsett, M. B.,** Structure and function of rat testis through pubescence, *Endocrinology,* 86, 1298, 1970.

58. **Pahnke, V. G., Leidenberger, F. R., and Kunzig, H. J.,** Correlation between hCG(LH)-binding capacity, Leydig cell number and secretory activity of rat testis throughout pubescence, *Acta Endocrinol.,* 79, 610, 1975.

59. **Pirke, K. M., Vogt, H. J., and Geiss, M.,** In vitro and in vivo studies on Leydig cell function in old rats, *Acta Endocrinol.,* 89, 393, 1978.

60. **Zirkin, B. R., Ewing, L. L., Kromann, N., and Cochran, R. C.,** Testosterone secretion by rat, rabbit, guinea pig, dog and hamster testes perfused in vitro; correlation with Leydig cell ultrastructure, *Endocrinology,* 107, 1867, 1980.

61. **Schapiro, B.,** Ist der Kryptorcidismus chirurgisch oder hormonell zu behandeln?, *Dtsch. Med. Wochenschr.,* 38, 38, 1931.

62. **Raynaud, A.,** Modification experimentale de la differention sexuelle des embryons des souris par action des hormones androgenes et oestrogenes, Herman et Cie, Paris, 1942.

63. **Jean, C.,** Croisance et structure des testicles cryptorchides chez les souris nees de mères traiteés a l'oestradiol pendant la gestation, *Ann. Endocrinol. (Paris),* 34, 669, 1973.

64. **Hadžiselimoviè, F. and Girard, J.,** Pathogenesis of cryptorchidism, *Hormone Res.,* 8, 76, 1977.

65. **Williams, R. G.,** Studies of living interstitial cells and pieces of seminiferous tubules in autogenous grafts of testis, *Am. J. Anat.,* 86, 343, 1950.

66. **Christensen, A. K. and Fawcett, D. W.,** The normal fine structure of testicular interstitial cells in guinea pigs, *J. Biophys. Biochem. Cytol.,* 9, 653, 1961.

67. **Charny, Ch. W., Conston, A. S., and Meranze, D. R.,** Development of the testis, *Fertil. Steril.,* 3, 461, 1952.

68. **Forest, M. G., Sizonenko, P. C., Cathiard, A. M., and Bertrand, J.,** Hypophyseal-gonadal function in humans during the first year of life. I. Evidence for testicular activity in early infancy, *J. Clin. Invest.,* 53, 819, 1974.

69. **Abraham, V. R., Born, H. J., Collischonn, G., Dericks-Tan, J. S., and Tanbert, H. D.,** Testosterone biosynthesis in spontaneous dystopic rat testes with genetic descensus disorder, *Endokrinologie,* 62, 368, 1973.

70. **Eik-Nes, K. B. E.,** Secretion of testosterone by the ectopic and the cryptorchid testis in the same dog, *Can. J. Physiol. Pharmacol.,* 44, 629, 1966.

71. **Gendrel, D., Job, J. C., and Roger, M.,** Reduced post-natal rise of testosterone in plasma of cryptorchid infants, *Acta Endocrinol.,* 89, 372, 1978.

72. **Atkinson, P. M., Epstein, M. T., and Rippon, A. E.,** Plasma gonadotropins and androgens in surgically treated cryptorchid patients, *J. Pediatr. Surg.,* 10, 27, 1975.

73. **Lipschutz, L. I., Caminos-Torres, R., Greenspan, C. S., and Snyder, P. J.,** Testicular function after orchiopexy for unilaterally undescended testis, *N. Engl. J. Med.,* 295, 15, 1976.

74. **Kodaira, T.,** Endocrinological studies on cryptorchidism, Part 3, Reference of endocrinological and histological changes due to HCG stimulation, *Jpn. J. Urol.,* 67, 807, 1976.

75. **Inaba, Y.,** Testicular-hypophyseal function observed in experimentally induced cryptorchidism in rat, *Jpn. J. Fertil. Steril.,* 25, 101, 1980.

Chapter 6

INFLUENCE OF CRYPTORCHIDISM ON LEYDIG CELL FUNCTION

Tom O. Abney and Brooks A. Keel

TABLE OF CONTENTS

I. INTRODUCTION

Experimental cryptorchidism was used as a method of studying testicular function as early as 1893.[1] Many of the structural changes which occur in the testis as a result of cryptorchidism were described years ago[2,3] and it has been known for some time that experimental cryptorchidism in the rat leads to severe damage to the spermatogenic process and rapid degeneration of the seminiferous epithelium.[4] It is also known that certain cell types appear to survive in cryptorchidism, although morphological alterations in these cells have been observed. Thus, spermatogonia, Sertoli cells, and Leydig cells are reported to remain intact.[5,6]

Various cryptorchid-induced changes have been described in the Sertoli cell, such as an incomplete maturation at puberty,[7] an increased number of Sertoli cells,[8] an increase in lipid droplets,[9] dilatation of the smooth endoplasmic reticulum,[10,11] and alterations of the inter-Sertoli cell junctional complexes.[10-12] It is now believed that alterations in Sertoli cell function may be one of the earliest effects of cryptorchidism.[11-14] Reduced production of androgen-binding protein (ABP) has been demonstrated in Sertoli cells of cryptorchid testes.[14-16] This decrease was shown to be a direct effect of cryptorchidism on the Sertoli cell since it was observed in the abdominal testis lacking germ cells. The demonstrations of decreased levels of inhibin[17,18] as well as aromatase activity in immature rats[18] provide further support for cryptorchid-induced Sertoli cell damage.

Concerning Leydig cell structure and function, Amatayakul et al.[19] reported that the cytoplasm increased and assumed a granular appearance after cryptorchidism. Clegg,[20] in fact, reported that a transient increase in the number of Leydig cells occurred within 21 d after cryptorchidism in the rat. Rager et al.,[21] measuring *in vitro* transformation of progesterone, reported a transient rise in testosterone 20 d after bilateral cryptorchidism. These results agree with the earlier findings of Clegg[22] and with the later reports that progesterone metabolism by the human undescended testis was not impaired.[23,24] In contrast to these findings, Inano and Tamaoki[25] reported a decrease in the enzymatic activities associated with androgen production in the abdominal testis of unilaterally cryptorchid rats. Similarly, a reduction in the testosterone content of the abdominal testis has been reported in unilaterally[26] and bilaterally cryptorchid[27] rats.

Kerr et al.[10] demonstrated that cryptorchidism resulted in hypertrophy of Leydig cells, yet a decreased responsiveness to human chorionic gonadotropin (hCG) treatment *in vivo.* There are numerous reports which substantiate the observation that cryptorchidism results in Leydig cell hypertrophy,[16,28] accompanied by decreased luteinizing hormone (LH) receptors[14,28,29] and an increased responsiveness to hCG *in vitro.*[16,29,30] It is possible that the elevated serum LH levels are responsible for the hypertrophy of Leydig cells, hyperresponsiveness to hCG stimulation *in vitro,* and the loss of LH receptors.

There is growing evidence for the existence of a relationship between Leydig cells and other testicular cell types (see Chapter 8). It has been postulated that Leydig cell function is controlled to some extent by factors (paracrine substances) from the seminiferous tubules (either germ cells or Sertoli cells). Thus, a series of complex cell-cell interactions are believed to exist, in which function by one cell type is influenced by one or several other cell types. Leydig cell function is conceivably regulated by germ cells, Sertoli cells, myoid cells, and/ or other cells. It follows, then, that cryptorchid-induced damage to the tubular compartment can alter this intercellular regulation. This raises the interesting question as to whether cryptorchid-induced changes in Leydig cell function are primary in nature or represent secondary alterations which result from altered paracrine regulatory mechanisms.

It was reported[31] that Leydig cell hypertrophy occurred around tubules in which spermatogenesis was disrupted, which suggests that tubules normally secrete factors that inhibit Leydig cell growth. Risbridger et al.[32] demonstrated that, in the cryptorchid rat, Leydig cell hypertrophy, hyperresponsiveness to hCG stimulation *in vitro,* and the loss of ^{125}I-labeled hCG binding to *in vitro* cannot be due to elevated serum LH levels, since serum LH levels failed to increase following unilateral cryptorchidism until 4 weeks. These authors also postulated that cryptorchidism decreased tubular-derived factors and consequently led to hypertrophy and hyperresponsiveness of Leydig cells. Recent evidence presented by other investigators[33,34] suggests that tubular (Sertoli) factors stimulate Leydig cell malfunction.[35,36] It remains to be determined whether the early changes in cryptorchid-induced Leydig cell function are the result of direct damage or represent secondary effects of altered paracrine substances.

In addition, recovery of testicular function and reversal of cryptorchid-induced damage through surgical repair (orchidopexy) have been the subjects of a limited number of studies to date. Most clinical studies indicate that orchidopexy should be performed prior to 6 to 8 years in humans,[37-39] otherwise irreversible damage occurs. Similar results have been reported in experimental animal models. Thus, diminished levels of prolactin (PRL) receptors[40] as well as numerous changes in Sertoli[16,41] and Leydig[16] cell functions are reversible only if orchidopexy is performed with 2 to 3 weeks after cryptorchidism. Furthermore, reversal of cryptorchid-induced damage is possible in immature, but not mature, rats.[16,40-42] Orchidopexy prior to sexual maturation appears to reverse the damage to the germinal epithelium and restore spermatogenesis. This is not the case in animals after sexual maturity. It is postulated therefore that recovery of the spermatogenic process is required for subsequent recovery of Sertoli and Leydig cell function. This also suggests that Sertoli and Leydig cell damage in cryptorchidism is associated with or is a consequence of spermatogenic damage.

Cryptorchidism also results in altered testicular blood flow,[43,44] and could lead to decreased metabolic clearance rate of steroids or a breakdown in the steroid-concentrating mechanisms of the pampiniform plexus. It is pertinent to note at this point that Turner et al.[45] demonstrated a partial disruption of the blood-testis barrier in the cryptorchid rat. As suggested previously, damage to the seminiferous epithelium may result in altered Leydig cell function. Sharpe[46] reported that cryptorchidism caused a delay in testicular capillary flow and a gross impairment of hCG uptake *in vivo* into interstitial tissue. A number of investigators have shown that LH[14,29] as well as PRL[40] binding capacity (i.e., receptors) are decreased in the cryptorchid testis. Increased serum gonadotropins, seen in bilateral cryptorchidism, accompanied by decreased steroid production might also reflect a down-regulation of testicular function, as suggested previously by de Kretser et al.[28] One or more of these mechanisms could explain how bilateral cryptorchidism leads to unchanged serum levels of testosterone and estradiol while the total testicular levels of these steroids remain reduced in the presence of increased gonadotropins.

In regard to the influence of cryptorchidism on serum hormone levels, conflicting results exist for practically all hormones measured thus far. For example, it is generally agreed that serum gonadotropin levels are increased in the cryptorchid rat;[19,47,48] however, several investigators have reported little or no change in follicle stimulating hormone (FSH)[49,50] and LH.[5,49,51] Recent evidence[52] indicates that cryptorchidism alters the relative and absolute amounts of the various LH isohormones produced by the pituitary, such that the most biologically active LH isohormone is increased (see Chapter 4). Serum testosterone levels in the cryptorchid rat are generally reported to be reduced[19,53,54] or unchanged.[7-48] Serum estradiol levels were demonstrated to be reduced in one investigation[54] and increased in another.[49] Bergh et al.[18] reported a decrease in estradiol synthesis (aromatase) as early as 6 h after cryptorchidism. To confound the issue, these discrepant results were obtained from different cryptorchid animal models of different ages with various durations of cryptorchidism (see Chapter 2 for discussion of animal models).

Concerning the possible role of estrogen in testicular function, Damber and Bergh[55] reported an increased concentration of estradiol in the cryptorchid testis. Evidence is accumulating which suggests that estrogens may act by a local feedback mechanism to regulate

Leydig cell activity. The Leydig cells have specific estrogen receptors[56] and *in vivo* administration of estrogens inhibited the response to LH and hCG stimulation;[57] it also reduced the number of hCG binding sites on the individual Leydig cell[58] and it directly inhibited some enzymes involved in the synthesis of testosterone.[59] Estrogen production, either by the tubular element[60] or by the Leydig cells,[61,62] may be sufficiently altered by cryptorchidism to affect a subsequent alteration of androgen synthesis and other Leydig cell processes. The bilaterally cryptorchid animal is a useful model for investigating testicular-pituitary relationships, altered function of Leydig cells, and the interactions between Leydig cells, germ cells, and Sertoli cells. The unilaterally cryptorchid animal serves as a unique model in that both the cryptorchid (abdominal) and eutopic (scrotal) testes are exposed to the same changes that may occur in the hormonal milieu as a result of cryptorchidism. This model thus allows for further investigation of possible compensatory or detrimental alterations in Leydig cell activity. Since cryptorchidism results in degeneration of the germinal epithelium and consequently in an *in situ* enrichment of Leydig cell concentration, the cryptorchid testis also serves as an excellent organ model from which Leydig cells can be purified for subsequent *in vitro* studies. Purification of Leydig cells from cryptorchid testes and subsequent examination of cellular functions *in vitro,* quantified per unit number of cells, can yield new information concerning the relationship between gonadotropin binding and steroid production. The studies outlined in this chapter include an investigation into the functional modifications of Leydig cells in bilaterally and unilaterally cryptorchid and eutopic testes.

II. STEROID PRODUCTION BY WHOLE TESTICULAR TISSUE

A. Influence of Bilateral Cryptorchidism

Over the course of the last decade, this laboratory has conducted studies on the influence of cryptorchidism on testicular function.[63-66] Initial studies utilized the bilaterally cryptorchid mature rat as a model to examine the steroidogenic capacity of whole testicular tissue *in vitro.*[64] In all the studies described here, mature male Sprague-Dawley rats were used. The animals were randomly divided into two groups, intact controls and animals which were made bilaterally cryptorchid.

To render the animals cryptorchid, the rats were anesthetized with sodium pentobarbital, a midline abdominal incision was made and both testes were drawn through the inguinal canal and sutured to the abdominal wall after severing the gubernaculum.[25,63] Sham operations were performed on the control group. At 7, 14, 21, and 28 d after surgery, five rats from each group were sacrificed and the testes were removed. Pooled testes from each group were placed in ice-cold medium-199 (M-199) buffer, decapsulated, and finely minced. Aliquots of 100 mg (wet weight) were placed in vials with 1.9 ml M-199 buffer; zero time samples were frozen immediately. For *in vitro* production of testosterone, triplicate samples were incubated for 3 h in a Dubnoff metabolic shaking incubator at 32°C with a 95% O_2-5% CO_2 atmosphere. Samples were frozen and stored at -20°C until assayed in subsequent RIAs.

The concentrations of testosterone, expressed as nanograms per 100 mg testicular tissue, at zero time and after a 3 h incubation are illustrated in Figure 1. The 3-hr values were corrected for the testosterone present in the respective zero time samples (t_3 - t_0) to yield the actual amount of testosterone produced *in vitro*. While the zero time concentrations in the control groups remained relatively constant throughout the study, the levels in the cryptorchid group increased significantly above the controls at 14 d ($p < 0.05$) and continued to rise above controls at 21 and 28 d ($p < 0.01$). Testosterone production *in vitro* exhibited a similar rise and was significantly increased above the control values at 14 d ($p < 0.05$) and 28 d ($p < 0.01$). The concentrations of estradiol, expressed as picograms per 100 mg testicular tissue, are depicted in Figure 2. The cryptorchid group exhibited a rise in testicular

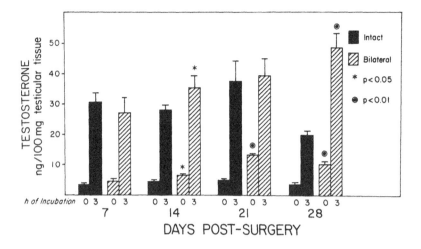

FIGURE 1.   Effects of bilateral cryptorchidism on testicular testosterone concentrations in the mature rat. Zero time concentrations and *in vitro* production after 3 h incubation of 100 mg minced testicular aliquots were determined. The values for *in vitro* testosterone production represent the total concentration after incubation minus the zero time concentration. Statistical analysis refers to a comparison between the cryptorchid and intact groups with the same incubation times on each day post surgery. (From Keel, B. A. and Abney, T. O., *Endocrinology*, 107, 1226, 1980. With permission.)

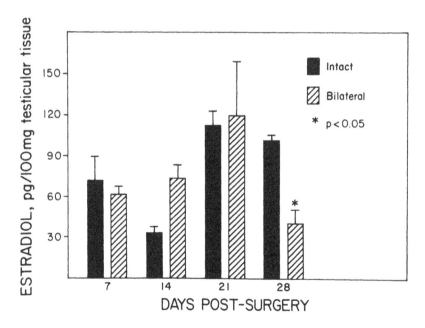

FIGURE 2.   Effects of bilateral cryptorchidism on testicular estradiol concentrations in the mature rat. Zero time estradiol concentrations of 100 mg minced testicular aliquots were determined. Statistical analysis refers to a comparison between the cryptorchid and intact groups on each day post surgery. (From Keel, B. A. and Abney, T. O., *Endocrinology*, 107, 1226, 1980. With permission.)

estradiol levels from 7 to 21 d, but these increases were insignificant when compared with the control groups. By 28 d, the testicular estradiol levels in the cryptorchid group were significantly decreased ($p < 0.05$) compared to the control levels.

The testicular content of testosterone, expressed as nanograms per testis, is shown in Table 1. These data indicate that bilateral cryptorchidism resulted in the reduction of both

Table 1
EFFECTS OF BILATERAL CRYPTORCHIDISM ON TESTICULAR
TESTOSTERONE CONTENT AND PRODUCTION

Incubation time	Day postsurgery	Control[a]	Bilateral[a]	% of control
Zero time (content)	7	56.9	36.1	63.5
	14	75.9	28.4	37.4
	21	81.3	53.2	65.5
	28	60.8	32.1	52.7
3 h (production)	7	502.1	221.4	44.1
	14	386.3	159.3	41.2
	21	611.1	158.4	25.9
	28	320.0	138.3	43.2

[a] The values for 3 h production represent the total content minus the zero time content. The mean testicular weight (grams per testis) was multiplied by the mean testosterone concentration (nanogram per gram) to obtain the above values, (nanogram per testis).

From Keel, B. A. and Abney, T. O., *Endocrinology*, 107, 1226, 1980. With permission.

Table 2
EFFECTS OF BILATERAL
CRYPTORCHIDISM ON TESTICULAR
ESTRADIOL CONTENT

Day postsurgery	Control[a]	Bilateral[a]	% of control
7	1166.0	507.8	43.6
14	550.6	334.5	60.7
21	1836.0	485.6	26.4
28	1628.9	123.0	7.6

[a] The mean testicular weight (grams per testis) was multiplied by the mean estradiol concentration (picogram per gram) to obtain the above values, expressed as content (picograms per testis).

From Keel, B. A. and Abney, T. O., *Endocrinology*, 107, 1226, 1980. With permission.

zero time testosterone levels and testosterone production compared to control groups. Seven days post surgery, a decrease in testosterone content was observed as a result of bilateral cryptorchidism. Similar decreases were exhibited by the bilateral groups at 14 through 28 d. The ability of the bilaterally cryptorchid testis to produce testosterone *in vitro* was also decreased when expressed per whole testis. The bilateral group demonstrated reductions in testosterone values at 7 through 28 d compared with controls. A corresponding decrease in testicular estradiol content, expressed as picograms per testis, was also demonstrated. As shown in Table 2, the level of testicular estradiol in the cryptorchid group, 7 d post surgery, decreased 56.4% compared to control levels. Analogous decreases of 39.3, 73.6, and 92.4% were seen 14, 21, and 28 d post surgery, respectively.

The total testicular content of testosterone (nanograms per testis) was reduced in the abdominal testis throughout this study as was the testicular production of testosterone per testis. An apparent discrepancy is noted if the content of testosterone is compared with the concentration of testosterone (nanograms per 100 mg testicular tissue). While the content of testosterone in the bilateral cryptorchid testis was reduced, an increase was observed when the data were expressed as a concentration. Several investigators[51,63,67] have reported that testicular weight decreases dramatically as a result of cryptorchidism. Because over 90% of the total testicular mass is composed of seminiferous tubules[68,69] which are damaged due to cryptorchidism[70] (see Chapter 9), a decrease in testicular mass would reflect the loss of germinal elements and an increase in the interstitial tissue volume in proportion to the other testicular components. Therefore, testosterone concentrations in the cryptorchid testis rose over intact control levels because the proportion of interstitial cells per unit weight of tissue in the abdominal testis was increased. If steroid production is taken as a marker of Leydig cell function, then the decrease in testosterone content would, at first glance, seem to indicate a detrimental influence of cryptorchidism in the testis. However, there is evidence which suggests that all functions of the Leydig cell are not adversely affected by cryptorchidism. The use of cytoplasmic estradiol receptor levels as a cell marker suggest, as will be discussed in more detail later in this chapter, that cryptorchidism results in little or no alteration in Leydig cell viability, at least in acute time periods.

Similar to the changes noted in testicular testosterone content, bilateral cryptorchidism caused a reduction in the testicular content of estradiol throughout this study. When the results are expressed as the concentration of estradiol, there appeared to be no significant difference between the control and bilateral groups through 21 d post surgery. The decrease in estradiol concentration seen in the bilateral group at 28 d cannot be explained. This difference could be due to animal variation, since a comparison of the cryptorchid groups (or intact) at different times post surgery showed some variation.

We have presented data which indicate that the testicular concentration of testosterone and estradiol and the production of testosterone *in vitro* per testis were decreased in the cryptorchid testis. Clearly, other mechanisms must be involved that would explain the discrepancy between unaltered steroid hormone levels in the serum and decreased levels in the testis. Cryptorchidism could result in an increased testicular blood flow[44,67] or breakdown in the steroid-concentrating mechanisms of the pampiniform plexus. Increased serum gonadotropins accompanied by decreased steroid production might also reflect a down-regulation of testicular function, as suggested by de Kretser et al.[28] Cryptorchidism might thereby lead to chronic desensitization of testicular steroidogenesis. One or more of these mechanisms could explain how bilateral cryptorchidism leads to unchanged serum levels of testosterone and estradiol while the total testicular levels of these steroids remain reduced.

B. Influence of Unilateral Cryptorchidism

The unilaterally cryptorchid animal offers a unique model for studying the effects of cryptorchidism on testicular function in that both the cryptorchid and eutopic testes are probably exposed to the same changes that might occur in the hormonal milieu as a result of the cryptorchidism. This animal model also allows the possible detection of any compensatory or detrimental changes which might occur in gonadal function. Indeed, a compensatory hyperplasia and hypertrophy of Leydig cells in the eutopic testis from the unilaterally cryptorchid rat have been reported.[71] However, definitive results concerning unilaterally cryptorchid-induced alterations in the testis and in the hormonal levels of these animals are still lacking. We have investigated the effects of unilateral cryptorchidism on testicular endocrine function using the mature rat as our model.

During the course of our studies, we observed no significant differences in the levels of serum testosterone between intact control and unilaterally cryptorchid animals.[65] However, we found that testicular content of testosterone was altered in the unilateral group. The content of testosterone, expressed as nanogram per testis, is shown in Figure 3. These data demonstrate a decrease in the testosterone content of the cryptorchid testis from 30.6 ± 3.3 ng at 7 d to 10.8 ± 0.3 ng at 28 d. This decrease below controls was statistically significant throughout the study ($p < 0.01$). The data also indicate a compensatory increase in testicular

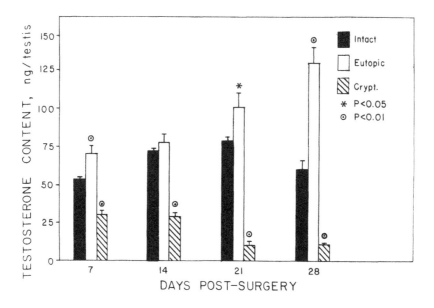

FIGURE 3.   Effects of unilateral cryptorchidism on testicular testosterone content, expressed as nanogram/testis. Statistical analysis refers to a comparison between the experimental and the control groups. (From Keel, B. A. and Abney, T. O., *Proc. Soc. Exp. Biol. Med.*, 166, 489, 1981. With permission.)

testosterone content of the eutopic testis above controls. Although an increase of 5% was not statistically significant at 14 d post surgery, significant increases above controls of 35% at 7 d ($p < 0.01$), 30% at 21 d ($p < 0.05$), and 113% at 28 d ($p < 0.01$) were detected.

In support of a possible compensatory change as a result of unilateral cryptorchidism, the data in Figure 3 indicate that, while the content of testosterone per testis in the cryptorchid testis was reduced below controls throughout this study, the content of testosterone per testis of the eutopic testis increased. By 28 d post surgery, the eutopic testis contained twice as much testosterone as the control testes and 13 times as much testosterone as the cryptorchid testis. Since the weights of the control and eutopic testes did not differ, these results suggest that the *in vivo* steroidogenic capacity of the eutopic testis was dramatically increased as a result of unilateral cryptorchidism. This increased capacity could be due to several factors, including hypertrophy of Leydig cells, increased steroidal enzymatic activity, and increased sensitivity to LH. First, hypertrophy of Leydig cells in the eutopic testis of unilaterally experimental[71] and congenital cryptorchid[72] rats has been reported. However, another study[26] failed to confirm this finding. Second, increases in 17α-hydroxylase[73] and Δ^5-3β-hydroxysteroid dehydrogenase[68] were observed in the eutopic testis when compared with the contralateral cryptorchid testis. Because these enzyme activities were not compared with those of intact controls, it is difficult to determine if a compensatory increase in steroidogenic enzymes existed in the eutopic testis as a result of unilateral cryptorchidism. Finally, it has been proposed that a compensatory mechanism in Leydig cells of the eutopic testis might involve an increase in sensitivity to LH stimulation.[26] It is conceivable, therefore, that unilateral cryptorchidism might increase the response of the eutopic testis to the normal circulating levels of LH through an increase in LH binding. This increased response would result in an increase in testosterone production, thus compensating for the decreased testicular content of testosterone exhibited by the cryptorchid testis.

III. PURIFICATION OF LEYDIG CELLS FROM CRYPTORCHID TESTES

A. Standardization of the Procedures

Leydig cells represent only about 3 to 5% of the cellular volume of the mature rat testis,[74]

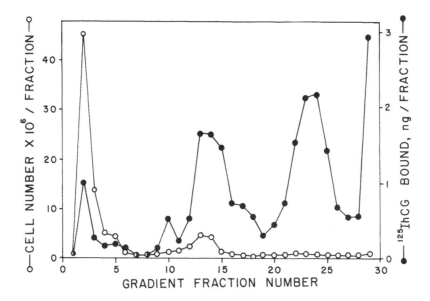

FIGURE 4. Specific ^{125}I-labeled hCG binding profile across an 11 to 27% equilibrated discontinuous metrizamide gradient. Populations I (fractions 11 to 15) and II (fractions 21 to 25) Leydig cells are represented by the two peaks of ^{125}I-labeled hCG. (From Abney, T. O. and Keel, B. A., *Arch. Androl.*, 17, 79, 1986. With permission.)

hence there exists the need to develop acceptable methods for isolation and purification of this important cell-type for endocrine studies. Numerous methods have been tested and adopted by investigators over the years, using various enzymes to digest the intact testis and obtain the interstitial tissue, and utilizing several gradient methods to purify the Leydig cells. Cells are usually identified as Leydig cells by ^{125}I-labeled hCG binding, gonadotropin responsive testosterone production, and histochemical staining for 3β-hydroxysteroid dehydrogenase.

Leydig cells can be separated by metrizamide density grandient centrifugation into two distinct populations (population I and II).[75,76] Different functional characteristics in terms of hCG binding and steroidogenic capacity have been attributed to the two populations,[77] thereby suggesting that Leydig cells may exist *in situ* as subpopulations with different functional roles. For example, the activity of the mitochondrial cytochrome P-450 side chain cleavage enzyme (P-450 SCC) differs between the two populations.[78] This provides further support for the existence of two populations *in situ* which differ in steroidogenic capacity. The question arises as to the influence of cryptorchidism on each of the different populations in terms of cell number, gonadotropin binding, and steroidogenic capacity.

Studies in this laboratory have employed a modified procedure similar to that described by O'Shaughnessy et al.[77] to obtain two distinct populations of Leydig cells. Briefly, collagenase dispersed interstitial cells (2 ml) were layered onto a 25-ml discontinuous gradient of metrizamide. The gradients were made up of 5 ml of 27%, 10 ml of 20%, and 10 ml of 11% metrizamide in M-199 The gradients were centrifuged at 3300 × *g* for 5 min and subsequently fractionated into 27 aliquots of 1 ml each. To assess the metrizamide gradient method for Leydig cell purification, equilibrated discontinuous gradients were used. Testicular interstitial cells were prepared from intact mature rat testes and incubated *in vitro* at 33°C for 1 hr with ^{125}I-labeled hCG. A second incubation was performed simultaneously with ^{125}I-labeled hCG plus a 1000-fold excess of unlabeled hCG. The incubations were cooled to 5°C and centrifuged to remove the cells from the incubation medium containing radioisotope. Each interstitial cell sample was resuspended in 2 ml M-199 and layered onto

Table 3

TESTOSTERONE PRODUCTION BY ISOLATED
LEYDIG CELLS FROM INTACT RATS

Cell fraction	ng/10^6 cells/3 h	Fold stimulation
Fraction 1—5		
Basal	0.30 ± 0.07[a]	—
+ hCG	0.51 ± 0.10[b]	1.7
+ dbcAMP	0.63 ± 0.15[b]	2.1
Population I		
Basal	7.19 ± 0.86[c]	—
+ hCG	83.95 ± 17.66[d]	10.9
+ dbcAMP	97.33 ± 22.65[d]	11.4
Population II		
Basal	12.84 ± 1.86[e]	—
+ hCG	166.37 ± 28.43[f]	13.5
+ dbcAMP	195.78 ± 40.30[f]	12.6

Note: Values with the same superscripts are statistically equivalent.
Responsiveness represents the stimulated (+ hCG or dbcAMP)
minus the unstimulated (basal) concentration of testosterone
produced *in vitro*. The values represent the mean ± SEM; n
= 10 experiments.

From Abney, T. O. and Keel, B. A., *Arch. Androl.*, 17, 79, 1986.
With permission.

a 25-ml gradient. Following centrifugation at 3300 × *g* for 5 min, the gradients were fractionated and the hCG-binding capacity and cell number in each of 27 × 1 ml fractions were determined. As shown in Figure 4, two major peaks of ^{125}I-labeled hCG binding were detected; cells in fractions 11 to 15 and 21 to 25 were designated as populations I and II, respectively. The hCG-binding profile shown in Figure 4 is almost identical to that reported by O'Shaughnessy et al.[77] for mature rat testis.

Cells from each population were further characterized as consisting of Leydig cells by other established criteria including androgen production and histochemical identification. As shown in Table 3, both population I and II cells were active in producing testosterone. In comparison, cells taken from the top of the gradient, fractions 1 to 5, produced very little testosterone *in vitro*. Basal testosterone production, expressed as ng/10^6 cells/3 h, was 7.2 and 12.8 for populations I and II, respectively, compared to 0.3 ng for fractions 1 to 5. *In vitro* responsiveness to 10 mIU hCG or 1.0 m*M* dibutyryl cyclic adenosine monophosphate (dbcAMP) was 10- to 13-fold above basal production in the populations as compared to 2-fold or less in fractions 1 to 5.

Histochemical analysis of cells from each fraction of the metrizamide gradient revealed that cells in populations I and II stained positive for 3β-hydroxysteroid dehydrogenase; cells from other regions of the gradient exhibited little or no staining capacity (Table 4). Populations I and II displayed 30 to 35% and 60 to 65% Leydig cells, respectively, while fractions 1 to 5 contain 1 to 2% stained cells. The presence of Leydig cells at the top of the gradient probably represents cell trapping at the uppermost interface during centrifugation.

B. Isolation of Cryptorchid Testis Leydig Cells

Preliminary studies on the influence of bilateral and unilateral cryptorchidism on Leydig cell function were performed using the mature (65 to 90 d) rat at 14 d post surgery as a model. The 14-d cryptorchid rat was chosen for the initial studies because many of the testicular alterations that occur as a result of cryptorchidism are detected at that time. The

Table 4

HISTOCHEMICAL STAINING OF ISOLATED LEYDIG CELLS FROM INTACT RAT TESTES

Cell fraction	Stained cells/total cells	% positive (Leydig cells)
Fraction 1—5	21/2056	0—1
Population I	527/1578	30—35
Population II	350/527	60—65

Note: Positive stained cells were categorized as Leydig cells. The values for percent positive stained cells represent the range which we obtained from replicate experiments. A minimum of 50 randomly selected fields were viewed under light microscopy at $400 \times$ magnification.

From Abney, T. O. and Carswell, L. S., *Mol. Cell. Endocrinol.*, 45, 157, 1986. With permission.

Table 5

RECOVERY OF TESTICULAR INTERSTITIAL CELLS AFTER COLLAGENASE DIGESTION USING EITHER THE STANDARD OR MODIFIED PROCEDURE

Digestion conditions	Testis	$(\times 10^6/\text{testis})$ $\overline{X} \pm$ SEM
Standard, 15 min	Intact control	125.9 ± 8.3
Modified, 25 min	Intact control	220.7 ± 27.9
Modified, 25 min	Bilateral cryptorchid	32.8 ± 2.8
Modified, 25 min	Unilateral cryptorchid	27.8 ± 3.2
Modified, 25 min	Eutopic cryptorchid	247.8 ± 17.4

Note: Each value is significantly different from the modified digest control cell number, $n = 7$ to 10 experiments. Eutopic refers to the unilateral scrotal testis.

standard procedures utilized in this laboratory for digestion of testes and isolation of interstitial cells, as described, were initially tested with cryptorchid testes and found to be inadequate.

Experiments were conducted to obtain satisfactory cell preparations by extending the digestion time from 15 to 25 min or longer. This and several other minor modifications failed to yield complete digestion of cryptorchid testes. Complete digestion was obtained through a 25-min digestion period in conjunction with pipetting the partial digests after the initial 15 min. This method proved to be reproducible and yielded homogenous tissue digests; control testes (both intact control and eutopic scrotal) were subjected to the same treatment so as to allow comparison of cell preparation.

As shown in Table 5, control tissue subjected to this modified digestion yielded 220 $\times$ 10^6 cells/testis in the "interstitial cell" preparation (post-collagenase) compared to 125 $\times$ 10^6 obtained with the standard 15 min digestion. Of particular interest were the dramatic decreases in cell numbers obtained from the bilateral and unilateral cryptorchid testis, 32.8 and 27.8 $\times$ 10^6 cells/testis, respectively. The eutopic (cryptorchid scrotal) testis yielded 247 $\times$ 10^6 cells/testis, comparable in number to the control. It thus appears that the modified digestion resulted in an approximate twofold increase in control interstitial cells compared to the shorter standard method. Second, the greatly reduced cell number in the cryptorchid animal probably reflects the severe damage and rapid degeneration of the seminiferous epithelium due to cryptorchidism.

At this point, we became interested in determining the influence of both 14- to 28-d cryptorchidism on Leydig cell isolation and recovery since subsequent experiments to assess Leydig cell function were to include both 14- and 28-d cryptorchid animals. To ascertain the nature of the cell preparations obtained from both control and cryptorchid testes, crude interstitial cell preparations were subsequently layered on 25 ml discontinuous, 11 to 27% metrizamide gradients and centrifuged as routinely done to obtain Leydig cell bands. An immediate technical problem which had to be resolved at this point concerned the numbers of cells from each group which were loaded onto the respective gradients. To load cells from an equivalent number of testes onto each gradient (e.g., one testis) would have required layering ($\geq 220 \times 10^6$ cells for both the control and eutopic groups, while layering only 30 to 47×10^6 cells per gradient for the cryptorchid groups. On the other hand, an attempt to load an equivalent number of cells (e.g., 200×10^6 cells) would have represented a disproportionate number of gonads per gradient between the controls and cryptorchid groups. Furthermore, the choice of either of these options (i.e., equivalent numbers of testes vs. cell number per gradient) involved yet another problem, inherent in any attempt to compare intact and cryptorchid testes. That is, an interstitial cell preparation from cryptorchid testes contains cell types that are probably different, in number and proportion, in comparison to that from intact testes. For example, an interstitial cell preparation from cryptorchid rat testes contains a smaller proportion of germ cell contaminants than does an interstitial cell preparation from intact testes.

Cognizant of this inherent difference, care was taken to load equivalent cell numbers (60 to 75×10^6 interstitial cells) for each group onto the respective gradients so as to avoid creating potential artifacts in cell banding during centrifugation which might be caused by either a large or variable cell number per gradient. This cell number represents approximately two testes per gradient for the cryptorchid groups and one fourth testis per gradient for control and eutopic testes. It was reasoned that cell numbers per gradient fraction could be subsequently standardized on a per testis basis, if deemed useful. Using this procedure, gradients were centrifuged, fractionated, and the cell numbers per fraction were obtained. The cell migration profiles obtained, expressed as cells $\times 10^6$ per gradient fraction, exhibited several interesting differences between groups. First, there were, as expected, relatively few cells present in fractions 1 to 7, the germ cell region of the gradient, in the cryptorchid groups as compared to the control and eutopic groups. A large proportion of interstitial cells (90%) sediment into this upper gradient region in intact testicular preparations. Second, we observed a higher number of population I cells from the cryptorchid testes compared to the scrotal testes when a fixed number of cells were layered on gradients. When the cell profiles were standardized and expressed as cells $\times 10^6$ per gradient fraction per testis, the only difference noted was a significant decrease ($P < 0.05$) in the 28-d unilateral population II cell profile when compared to either the control or the 14-d unilateral population II cell numbers. The cell numbers from population I (fractions 11 to 15) and population II (fractions 21 to 25) were each pooled, computed, and standardized to the number of cells isolated on a per testis basis, as shown in Table 6. These data indicate that, although recoverable interstitial cell number was greatly reduced in the bilateral and unilateral cryptorchid testes (Table 5), there was little difference in the cell numbers isolated in the Leydig cell regions of the gradients. The capacity of these various purified Leydig cell preparations to bind ^{125}I-labeled hCG and to respond to gonadotropin and dbcAMP stimulation of testosterone production will be discussed in the next section of this chapter.

IV. PROPERTIES OF PURIFIED LEYDIG CELLS FROM THE CRYPTORCHID RAT TESTES

To ascertain the capacity of the Leydig cells isolated from cryptorchid testes to bind gonadotropin hormone, the specific binding of ^{125}I-labeled hCG across the gradient from

Table 6
RECOVERY OF LEYDIG CELLS USING METRIZAMIDE GRADIENT CENTRIFUGATION

Group	Population I		Population II	
	Duration of cryptorchidism			
	14 d	28 d	14 d	28 d
Control	5.69 ± 1.3	6.83 ± 0.98	2.68 ± 0.47	2.77 ± 0.56
Bilateral	7.8 ± 0.5	8.7 ± 1.59	2.08 ± 0.09	2.18 ± 0.10
Unilateral	6.28 ± 0.7	4.98 ± 1.5	2.09 ± 0.13	1.42 ± 0.14[a]
Eutopic	7.09 ± 1.02	8.2 ± 1.97	1.97 ± 0.47	2.47 ± 0.66
$\overline{X}$	6.72	7.18	2.21	2.21

Note: Above values represent the $\overline{X}$ ± SEM (10^6 cells/testis). These values were obtained by calculating the (cells/population) ÷ (testes/population) to yield cells/testis.

[a] Significantly different from both the respective control ($p <0.05$) and the 14 d unilateral ($p <0.05$)

14- and 28-d cryptorchid rats, expressed as disintegrations per minute (dpm) per testis per gradient was determined. No changes in hCG binding by population I Leydig cells from 14-d cryptorchid testes were observed when compared to controls. However, the amount of hCG bound by population I cells from eutopic testes was slightly higher when compared to the controls. In population II, although not significant, the binding in the cryptorchid testes was decreased from that of the control and eutopic cell preparations.

The peaks of ^{125}I-labeled hCG binding in fractions 11 to 15 and 21 to 25 from 11 to 27% discontinuous metrizamide gradients correspond to the peaks of cells previously designated by this laboratory and other investigators as population I and II Leydig cells. The dpms per pooled population, shown in Figure 5, illustrate that the binding in population I was relatively unaffected by cryptorchidism while the binding in population II was beginning to decrease. The specific binding of ^{125}I-labeled hCG by 28-d cryptorchid testes was similar to that seen at 14 d in population I. That is, no effect of cryptorchidism on the amount of hCG bound was seen in population I. Population II Leydig cells from bi- and unilateral cryptorchid testes exhibited significantly decreased ($p <0.05$) specific binding of hCG when compared to the respective controls. These results are depicted in Figure 6. Again, the decrease in hCG bound by population II from the cryptorchid testes is evident.

Having established that cryptorchidism had a detrimental effect on hCG binding by population II cells, particularly at 28 d, it then became of interest to investigate the steroidogenic capacity of these cell preparations. *In vitro* incubations utilizing Leydig cells from 14-d cryptorchid testes and a single dose of hCG (10 mIU) or dbcAMP (1.0 m*M*) yielded results which are illustrated in Figure 7. The amount of testosterone produced by the bi- and unilateral testes was decreased significantly ($p <0.01$) from the control values in both populations I and II. Testosterone production by Leydig cells from eutopic testes 14 d post surgery was not different from control values in either population. A similar study using testes from 28-d cryptorchid rats was performed (Figure 8). The production of testosterone by unilateral testes was significantly decreased below the control in both populations ($p <0.05$). In contrast, hCG-stimulated testosterone production from bilateral testes was decreased, but not significantly below control values in population I while population II Leydig cells from bilateral testes also did not exhibit any significant change in the amount of testosterone produced compared to controls. Testosterone production by Leydig cells from eutopic testes at 28 d was slightly, though significantly ($p <0.05$), increased in population I cells. Population II cells from the eutopic testis exhibited no change from control values.

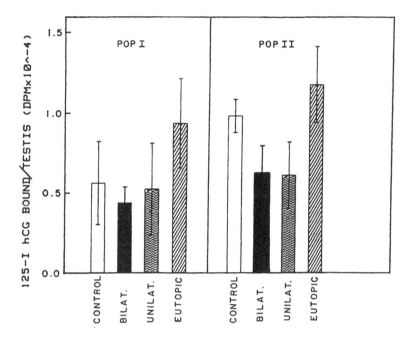

FIGURE 5. Interstitial cells from control, 14 d bilateral and unilateral cryptorchid and eutopic testes were incubated with ^{125}I-labeled hCG as described, centrifuged on metrizamide gradients, and the gradients were fractionated and counted. The values represent the specific binding of hCG from the pooled populations I (11 to 15) and II (21 to 25) of the various experimental groups. Specific binding has been corrected to a per testis basis.

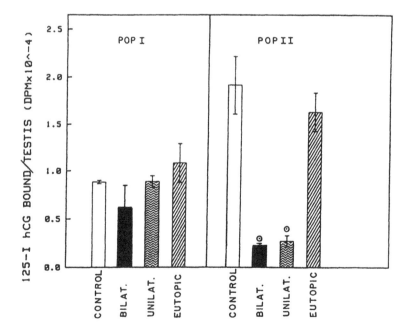

FIGURE 6. Interstitial cells from control, 28 d bilateral and unilateral cryptorchid and eutopic testes were incubated with ^{125}I-labeled hCG as described, centrifuged on metrizamide gradients, and the gradients were fractionated and counted. The values represent the specific binding of hCG from the pooled populations I (11 to 15) and II (21 to 25) of the various experimental groups. Specific binding has been corrected to a per testis basis.

107

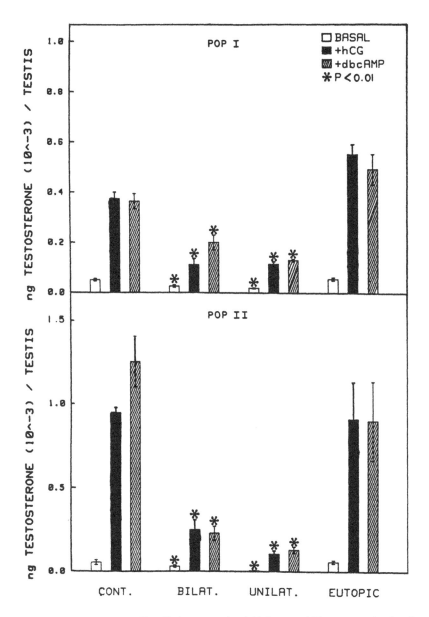

FIGURE 7. Isolated Leydig cells from control and 14-d cryptorchid testes were incubated for 3 h at 34°C in the absence or presence of hCG (10 mIU) or dbcAMP (1.0 m*M*). The amount of testosterone produced per population was standardized to a per testis basis. The values represent the mean ± SEM of three experiments with triplicate determinations within each.

These above data were obtained with a single dose of either hCG or dbcAMP. These concentrations of hormones are known from studies in our laboratory to yield maximum *in vitro* stimulation of testosterone production in testicular tissue minces or Leydig cell preparations from mature intact rats. There is evidence that cryptorchidism leads to decreased LH receptors and results in a hyperresponsive stimulation of steroidogenesis. It is, therefore, possible that the dose responses to hCG and dbcAMP would be different for Leydig cells from intact and cryptorchid testes. Dose response experiments were performed utilizing a wide range of hCG concentrations (0 to 200 mIU) in an attempt to characterize the responsiveness of each Leydig cell population. An increase in testosterone production *in vitro* in

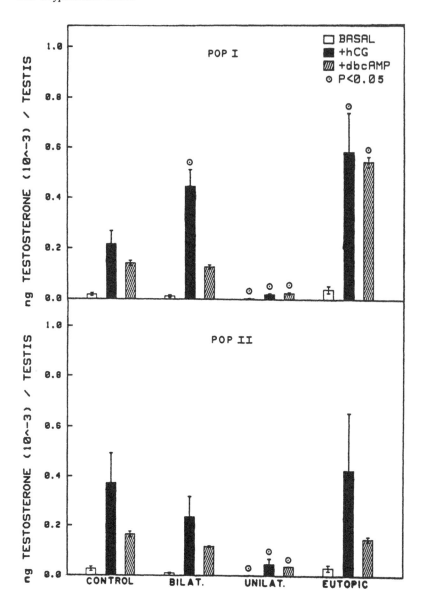

FIGURE 8. Isolated Leydig cells from control and 28-d cryptorchid testes were incubated for 3 h at 34°C in the absence or presence of hCG (10 mIU) or dbcAMP (1.0 m*M*). The amount of testosterone produced per population of Leydig cells was standardized to a per testis basis. The values represent the mean ± SEM of three experiments with triplicate determinations within each.

response to increasing concentrations of hCG was seen among all four groups (controls, bilateral, unilateral, and eutopic) in both populations at the two times studied, 14 and 28 d postsurgery. The 14-d studies (Figure 9) revealed that even though the amount of testosterone produced by the cryptorchid testis increased with increasing doses of hCG, the levels of testosterone production still remained below those of control and eutopic levels in both populations. The amount of testosterone produced by the eutopic was not different from that produced by control testes. The *in vitro* incubations utilizing 28-d cryptorchid testes, as illustrated in Figure 10, show that the bilateral and eutopic population I Leydig cells at the higher doses of hCG (10, 50, and 200 mIU) produced significantly ($p < 0.05$) higher amounts

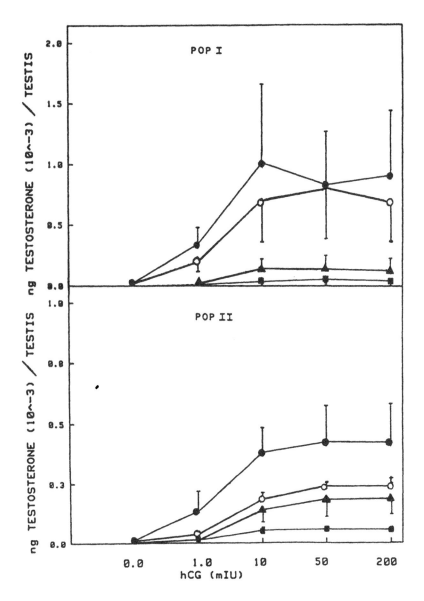

FIGURE 9.   Isolated Leydig cells from control (●), 14 d bilateral (▲), 14 d unilateral (■) and eutopic (○) was incubated *in vitro* in the absence or the presence of increasing doses of hCG. Testosterone production was standardized to a per testis basis. The values represent the mean ± SEM of three experiments with triplicate determinations within each.

of testosterone than the control. The unilateral cryptorchid cells produced significantly (p <0.05) less testosterone than controls in both populations in response to all concentrations of hCG.

This study demonstrates that the testes from 14- to 28-d cryptorchid rats show dramatic differences in their *in vitro* steroidogenic secretory capacity compared to testes from control rats. The data from the 14-d cryptorchid dose-response experiments demonstrate that the population I and II Leydig cells from cryptorchid testes are less sensitive and less responsive to hCG compared to controls. The dose-response experiments confirm the earlier experiments performed with a single concentration of hCG or dbcAMP; compare Figure 7 with Figure 9 for the 14-d experiments.

The 28-d dose-response study yielded results slightly different from those of the 14-d

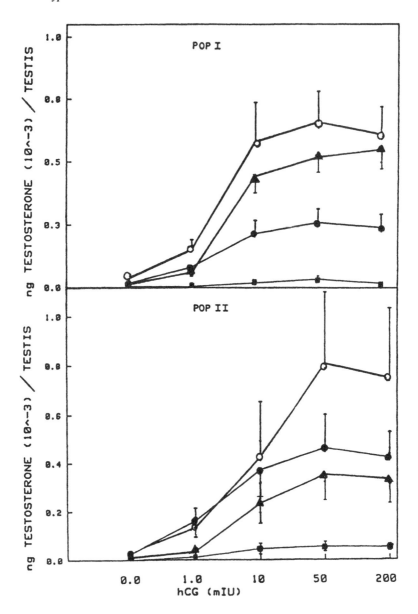

FIGURE 10.   Isolated Leydig cells from control (●), 28 d bilateral (▲), 28 d unilateral (■) and eutopic (○) were incubated *in vitro* in the absence or presence of increasing doses of hCG. The values represent the mean ± SEM from four experiments with triplicate determinations within each.

experiment. The unilateral cryptorchid Leydig cells from both populations remained less sensitive and less responsive to stimulation. While the eutopic cells were as sensitive or more and were hyperresponsive to stimulation by hCG when compared to control, the hyperresponsiveness of the eutopic testes was not seen in the 14-d study but is obvious at 28 d post surgery (Figure 10). The eutopic testes appeared to be compensating for the lack of testosterone production by the unilateral cryptorchid testes. The hCG dose response data at both 14 and 28 d for both populations I and II, clearly reveal that Leydig cells from the unilateral cryptorchid testis exhibited the most dramatic decrease in sensitivity and responsiveness to stimulation. In addition, uniscrotal (eutopic) Leydig cells were either equal to or greater than the controls, particularly at 28 d post surgery. In contrast, Leydig cells from

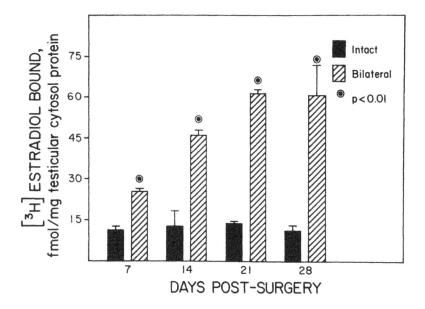

FIGURE 11. Effects of bilateral cryptorchidism on the levels of testicular cytoplasmic estradiol receptor, determined *in vitro* and analyzed by Scatchard plots. The data were corrected for nonspecific binding. Each value represents the mean ± SEM from two experiments. Statistical analysis refers to a comparison between the cryptorchid and intact groups on each day post surgery. (From Keel, B. A. and Abney, T. O., *Endocrinology*, 107, 1226, 1980. With permission.)

the bilateral group appeared to recover their steroidogenic capacity at 28 d, exhibiting production levels equal to or greater than controls. Summarizing the results obtained in these studies:

1.   The amount of hCG bound by the cryptorchid testis at both 14 and 28 d post surgery in population I was not different from controls, while hCG binding capacity in population II decreased significantly at 28 days.
2.   The amount of testosterone produced by the unilateral testis (population I and II Leydig cells) was dramatically decreased from controls at both 14 and 28 d.

V. EFFECTS OF CRYTORCHIDISM ON ESTROGEN-BINDING CAPACITY IN THE TESTIS

Considering that cryptorchidism alters Leydig cell morphology and testosterone synthesis and that estradiol exerts an effect on Leydig cell metabolism, it was of interest to examine the effects of uni- and bilateral cryptorchidism on the estradiol-binding capacity of the testis.[64-65] As in previous studies, adult rats were made either bi- or unilaterally cryptorchid for a period of 7, 14, 21, or 28 d; intact sham-operated rats served as controls. As shown in Figure 11, bilateral cryptorchidism resulted in a marked increase in estradiol binding compared with controls. The cytoplasmic estrogen receptor levels, expressed as femtomole of ^{3}H-estradiol per milligram cytosol protein, for the control and bilateral groups at 7 d were 11.1 ± 0.8 and 25.6 ± 0.9, respectively. This twofold increase above controls was maintained by the bilateral group 14 d postsurgery and rose further at 21 and 28 d to a fourfold increase in binding.

The possibility that bilateral cryptorchidism could alter the binding properties of the receptor was considered; the association constant (K_a) at equilibrium was essentially un-

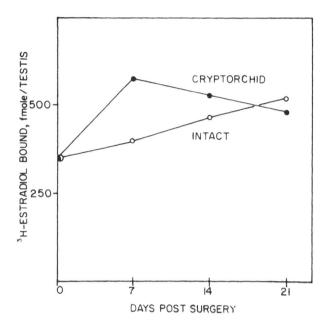

FIGURE 12.   Specific binding of estradiol/testis from intact control and
bilaterally cryptorchid rats. The cytosols were assessed for estradiol binding
in vitro. These values were computed by using the mean values (estradiol
bound/milligram cytosol protein) × (milligram cytosol protein/gram tissue) × (gram tissue/testis). Specific estradiol binding by intact control
cytosol was 16 ± 1.1 fmol/mg protein; a mean of 20.5 ± 0.5 mg cytosol
protein/gram tissue was obtained. Each value is the mean of duplicate
experiments using pooled testicular tissue. (From Abney, T. O., Grier,
H., and Mahesh, V. B., *Endocrinology,* 101, 975, 1977. With permission.)

changed for each of the cytosol receptor preparations. An average value for the K_a of 3×10^{10} M^{-1} was obtained, illustrating that the binding affinity of the receptor was not altered
by cryptorchidism. However, the number of binding sites per milligram cytosol protein
increased dramatically in the 21-d experimental period. This increase reflects the cellular
changes that occurred after cryptorchidism and not alterations in receptor binding properties.

The content of cytoplasmic estradiol receptors, expressed per testis, revealed a pattern
that was different from the observed alteration in receptor concentration (per milligram
cytosol protein) described earlier. Figure 12 illustrates that the estradiol receptor content of
the cryptorchid testis increased above controls in the 1st week after surgery but returned to
control levels by the 3rd week. All the parameters measured in this study, expressed as a
percent of controls values, allows a comparison of the increase in estradiol binding with the
diminution of testicular weight. Estradiol binding per milligram cytosol protein was greatly
increased above controls as early as day 7 following cryptorchidism and rose still further
by days 14 and 21. This rise was greater than the corresponding decrease in testis weight
and reflects primarily the loss in germinal epithelium and the subsequent increase in the
interstitial tissue volume in proportion to the other testicular components. When expressed
on a per testis basis, the data indicate that the estradiol receptor content did not decrease as
a result of bilateral cryptorchidism. Using estradiol-binding levels as a cell marker, the above
data would suggest that little or no change occurred in the viability of the Leydig cell
population.

Unilateral cryptorchidism resulted in similar changes in the estradiol-binding capacity of
the abdominal testis. As depicted in Figure 13, unilateral cryptorchidism resulted in a marked
increase in the cytoplasmic estradiol-binding capacity by cryptorchid testes when compared

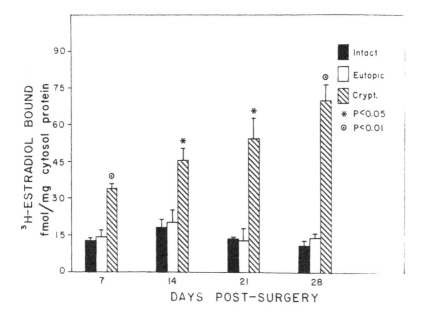

FIGURE 13. Effects of unilateral cryptorchidism on the levels of testicular cytoplasmic estrogen receptor. The cytoplasmic estradiol binding capacity, expressed as femtomole ³H-estradiol bound/milligram testicular cytosol protein, was determined *in vitro* and analyzed by Scatchard plots. The data were corrected for nonspecific binding. Each value represents the mean ± SEM from two experiments each utilizing pooled tissue. Statistical analysis refers to a comparison between the experimental and the control groups. (From Keel, B. A. and Abney, T. O., *Proc. Soc. Exp. Biol. Med.*, 166, 489, 1981. With permission.)

with the controls. This represents a threefold increase above controls at 7 and 14 d and was further increased to fourfold at 21 d and sixfold at 28 d. The cytoplasmic estrogen receptor-binding capacity of the eutopic testes was found to be equivalent to that of the controls at all time points. Testicular content of cytoplasmic estradiol receptor, expressed per testis, is presented in Table 7. These data reveal that estrogen-binding capacity in the controls, although somewhat variable, did not change significantly throughout the study. Receptor content in both the eutopic and cryptorchid testes did not differ significantly from the mean control value.

Evidence which suggests that all functions of the Leydig cells were not affected by unilateral cryptorchidism is provided by the fact that the concentrations of the cytoplasmic estradiol receptor in cryptorchid testes were increased above controls at all time points. This increase in binding capacity would reflect an increase in the Leydig cell proportion due to the loss of the germinal epithelium. Using estradiol-binding capacity as one parameter of cell function, this would suggest that little change had occurred in the viability of the Leydig cell population in the unilaterally cryptorchid testis. Further, when the estradiol-binding data were expressed per organ (Table 7), no differences were detected among the various groups. This observation suggests that the actual number of Leydig cells per testis were not increased. Further research is needed in this area to determine the effects of cryptorchidism on Leydig cell number and viability, and to delineate the mechanisms by which cryptorchidism alters testicular function.

ACKNOWLEDGMENTS

This investigation was supported, in part, by funds from NIH (R01-HD16983), NSF (PCM-8109847), and BRSG (2S07RR05365-19). BAK was a recipient of an NIH Training Grant (5T32HD 07110-04) while a student.

Table 7
EFFECTS OF UNILATERAL CRYPTORCHIDISM ON CYTOPLASMIC ESTRADIOL BINDING CAPACITY, FEMTOMOLES OF ^{3}H-ESTRADIOL BOUND PER TESTIS[a]

Day post surgery	Control	Eutopic	Cryptorchid
7	336	431	453
14	560	668	449
21	441	494	377
28	369	453	418
$\bar{X}^b \pm$ SE	426 ± 50	511 ± 53	424 ± 18

[a] The values were computed by using the mean values: (estradiol bound/milligram cytosol protein) × (mg cytosol protein/gram tissue) × (gram tissue/testis). A mean of 20.5 ± 0.5 mg cytosol protein/gram tissue was obtained over a wide range of experiments.

[b] Refers to the mean of each group for the 28 d of study.

From Keel, B. A. and Abney, T. O., *Proc. Soc. Exp. Biol. Med.,* 166, 489, 1980. With permission.

REFERENCES

1. **Griffiths, J.,** The structural changes in the testicle of the dog when it is replaced within the abdominal cavity, *J. Anat. Physiol.,* 27, 482, 1893.
2. **Moore, C. R.,** Properties of the gonads as controllers of somatic and physical characteristics. IV. Testicular reactions in experimental cryptorchidism, *Am. J. Anat.,* 34, 269, 1924.
3. **Steinberger, E. and Nelson, W. O.,** Effect of hypophysectomy, cryptorchidism, estrogen and androgen upon the level of hyaluronidase in the rat testis, *Endocrinology,* 56, 429, 1955.
4. **Nelson, W. O.,** Some factors involved in the control of the gametogenic and endocrine functions of the testis, *Cold Spring Harbor Symp. Q. Biol.,* 5, 123, 1937.
5. **Altwein, J. E. and Gittes, R. F.,** Effects of cryptorchidism and castration on FSH and LH levels in the adult rat, *Invest. Urol.,* 10, 167, 1972.
6. **Chowdhury, A. K. and Steinberger, E.,** The influence of a cryptorchid milieu on the initiation of spermatogenesis of the rat, *J. Reprod. Fertil.,* 29, 173, 1972.
7. **Hadziselemovic, F.,** Cryptorchidism, ultrastructure of normal and cryptorchid testis development, *Adv. Anat. Embryol. Cell Biol.,* 53(Fasc.), 3, 1, 1977.
8. **Clegg, E. J.,** Studies on artificial cryptorchidism: morphological and quantitative changes in the Sertoli cells of the rat testes, *J. Endocrinol.,* 26, 567, 1963.
9. **Leeson, T. S. and Leeson, C. R.,** Experimental cryptorchidism in the rat, a light and electron microscope study, *Invest. Urol.,* 8, 127, 1970.
10. **Kerr, J. B., Rich, K. A., and de Kretser, D. M.,** Effects of experimental cryptorchidism on the ultrastructure and function of the Sertoli cell and pretibular tissue of the rat testis, *Biol. Reprod.,* 21, 823, 1979.
11. **Bergh, A.,** Early morphological changes in abdominal testes in immature unilaterally cryptorchid rats, *Int. J. Androl.,* 6, 73, 1983.
12. **Aumuller, G., Hartman, K., Giers, U., and Schenk, B.,** Fine structure of the Sertoli cells of the testis in experimental cryptorchidism, *Int. J. Androl.,* 3, 301, 1980.
13. **Bergh, A.,** Morphological signs of a direct effect of experimental cryptorchidism on the Sertoli cells in rats irradiated as fetuses, *Biol. Reprod.,* 24, 145, 1981.
14. **Jegou, B., Risbridger, G. P., and de Kretser, D. M.,** Effects of experimental cryptorchidism on testicular function in adult rats, *J. Androl.,* 4, 88, 1983.

15. **Hagenas, L. and Ritzen, E. M.,** Impaired Sertoli cell function in experimental cryptorchidism in the rat, *Mol. Cell Endocrinol.,* 4, 25, 1976.
16. **Jegou, B., Peake, R. A., Irby, D. C., and de Kretser, D. M.,** Effects of the induction of experimental cryptorchidism and subsequent orchidopexy on testicular function in immature rats, *Biol. Reprod.,* 30, 179, 1984.
17. **Au, C. L., Robertson, D. M., and de Kretser, D. M.,** In vitro bioassay of inhibin in testes of normal and cryptorchid rats, *Endocrinology,* 112, 239, 1983.
18. **Bergh, A., Damber, J. E., and Ritzen, M.,** Early signs of Sertoli and Leydig cell dysfunction in the abdominal testes of immature unilaterally cryptorchid rats, *Int. J. Androl.,* 7, 398, 1984.
19. **Amatayukul, K., Ryan, R., Uozomi, T., and Albert, A.,** A reinvestigation of testicular-anterior pituitary relationships in the rat, *Endocrinology,* 88, 872, 1971.
20. **Clegg, E. J.,** Further studies on artificial cryptorchidism: quantitative changes in the interstitial cells of the rat testis, *J. Endocrinol.,* 24, 433, 1961.
21. **Rager, K., Arnold, E., Hauschild, A., and Gupta, D.,** Effect of bilateral cryptorchidism on the *in vitro* transformation of progesterone by testicular tissue at different stages of sexual maturation, *J. Steroid Biochem.,* 6, 1537, 1975.
22. **Clegg, E. J.,** Some effects of artificial cryptorchidism on the accessory reproduction organs of the rat, *J. Endocrinol.,* 20, 210, 1960.
23. **Lackgren, G. and Berg, A. A.,** The effects of hCG-treatment on *in vitro* metabolism of progesterone by the human undescended pre-pubertal testis, *Int. J. Androl.,* 6, 414, 1983.
24. **Lackgren, G. and Berg, A. A.,** *In vitro* metabolism of progesterone by the human undescended testis, *Int. J. Androl.,* 6, 423, 1983.
25. **Inano, H. and Tamaoki, B. I.,** Effects of experimental bilateral cryptorchidism on testicular enzymes related to androgen formation, *Endocrinology,* 83, 1074, 1968.
26. **Bergh, A. and Damber, J. E.,** Morphometric and functional investigation on the Leydig cells in experimental unilateral cryptorchidism in the rat, *Int. J. Androl.,* 1, 549, 1978.
27. **Hadziselimovic, F. and Girard, J.,** Pathogenesis of cryptorchidism, *Horm. Res.,* 8, 76, 1977.
28. **de Kretser, D. M., Sharpe, R. M., and Swanston, I. A.,** Alterations in steroidogenesis and human chorionic gonadotropin binding in the cryptorchid rat testis, *Endocrinology,* 105, 135, 1979.
29. **Huhtaniemi, I., Bergh, A., Nikula, H., and Damber, J. E.,** Differences in the regulation of steroidogenesis and tropic hormone receptors between the scrotal and abdominal testes of unilaterally cryptorchid adult rats, *Endocrinology,* 115, 550, 1984.
30. **Sharpe, R. M., Cooper, I., and Doogan, D. G.,** Increase in Leydig cell responsiveness in the unilaterally cryptorchid rat testis and its relationship to the intratesticular levels of testosterone, *J. Endocrinol.,* 102, 319, 1984.
31. **Aoki, A. and Fawcett, D. W.,** Is there a local feedback from the seminiferous tubules affecting activity on the Leydig cells?, *Biol. Reprod.,* 19, 144, 1978.
32. **Risbridger, G. P., Kerr, J. B., and de Kretser, D. M.,** Evaluation of Leydig cell function and gonadotropin binding in unilateral and bilateral cryptorchidism: evidence for local control of Leydig cell function by the seminiferous tubule, *Biol. Reprod.,* 24, 534, 1981.
33. **Main, S. J. and Setchell, B. P.,** Responsiveness of the pituitary gland to androgens and of the testis to gonadotropins following damage to the spermatogenesis in rats, *J. Endocrinol.,* 87, 445, 1980.
34. **Grotjan, H. E. and Heindel, J. J.,** Effect of spent media from Sertoli cell cultures on *in vitro* testosterone production by rat testicular interstitial cells, *N.Y. Acad. Sci.,* The Cell Biology of the Testis, (Abstr.) 2, 1981.
35. **Bergh, A.,** Paracrine regulation of Leydig cells by the seminiferous tubules, *Int. J. Androl.,* 6, 57, 1983.
36. **Bergh, A. and Damber, J. E.,** Local regulation of Leydig cells by the seminiferous tubules, Effects of short-term cryptorchidism, *Int. J. Androl.,* 7, 409, 1984.
37. **Levin, A. and Sherman, J. O.,** The undescended testis, *Surg. Gynecol. Obstet.,* 136, 473, 1973.
38. **Anoussakis, C., Liakakos, D., Kirburis, J., Papaspyrou, P., and Doulas, N. L.,** Effect of surgical repair of cryptorchidism on endocrine testicular function, *J. Pediatr.,* 103, 919, 1983.
39. **Duvie, S. O. A.,** Histological changes in the testis following adult orchidopexy for unilateral cryptorchidism, *Arch. Androl.,* 12, 231, 1984.
40. **Hochberg, Z., Amit, T., Youdim, M. B. H., and Bar-Maor, J. A.,** Prolactin binding by testes of unilaterally cryptorchid rats: the effects of hCG, testosterone, prolactin and orchidopexy, *Acta Endocrinol.,* 102, 144, 1983.
41. **Jahnsen, T., Karpa, B., Attramadal, H., Ritzen, M., and Hansson, V.,** Changes in isoproterenol-stimulated adenylate cyclase activity in rat testicular tissue during cryptorchidism and after orchidopexy, *J. Reprod. Fertil.,* 70, 443, 1984.
42. **Jegou, B., Laws, A. O., and de Kretser, D. M.,** The effects of cryptorchidism and subsequent orchidopexy in testicular function in adult rats, *J. Reprod. Fertil.,* 69, 137, 1983.

43. **Damber, J. E., Bergh, A., and Janson, P. O.,** Testicular blood flow and testosterone concentrations in the spermatic venous blood in rats with experimental cryptorchidism, *Acta Endocrinol. (Copenhagen),* 88, 611, 1978.

44. **Gomes, D., Kein, N. D., and Hamlin, R. L.,** Testicular blood flow and testosterone secretion rates in normal and cryptorchid rats, *Physiologist,* 19, 208, 1976.

45. **Turner, T. T., D'Addario, D. A., Forrest, J. B., and Howards, S. S.,** The effects of experimental cryptorchidism on the entry of [³H]-inulin and [³H]-horseradish peroxidase in the lumen of the rat seminiferous tubules, *J. Androl.,* 3, 178, 1982.

46. **Sharpe, R. M.,** Impaired gonadotropin uptake *in vivo* by the cryptorchid testis, *J. Reprod. Fertil.,* 67, 379, 1983.

47. **Gupta, D., Rager, K., Zarzycki, J., and Eichner, M.,** Levels of luteinizing hormone, follicle-stimulating hormone, testosterone, and dihydrotestosterone in the circulation of sexually maturing intact male rats and after orchidectomy and experimental bilateral cryptorchidism, *J. Endocrinol.,* 66, 183, 1975.

48. **Gomes, W. R. and Jain, S. K.,** Effects of unilateral and bilateral castration and cryptorchidism on serum gonadotropins in the rat, *J. Endocrinol.,* 68, 191, 1976.

49. **Jones, T. M., Anderson, W., Fung, V. S., Landau, R. L., and Rosenfield, R. L.,** Experimental cryptorchidism in the adult male rats: histological and hormonal sequelae, *Anat. Rec.,* 189, 1, 1977.

50. **Steinberger, E. and Chowdhury, M.,** Control of pituitary FSH in male rats, *Acta Endocrinol. (Copenhagen),* 76, 235, 1974.

51. **Swerdloff, R. A., Walsh, P. C., Jacobs, H. S., and Odell, W. D.,** Serum LH and FSH during sexual maturation in the male rat: effect of castration and cryptorchidism, *Endocrinology,* 88, 120, 1971.

52. **Keel, B. A. and Grotjan, H. E., Jr.,** Influence of bilateral cryptorchidism on rat pituitary luteinizing hormone charge microheterogeneity, *Biol. Reprod.,* 32, 83, 1985.

53. **Lloyd, B. J.,** Plasma testosterone and accessory sex glands in normal and cryptorchid rats, *J. Endocrinol.,* 54, 285, 1972.

54. **Hall, R. W. and Gomes, W. R.,** The effect of artificial cryptorchidism on serum oestrogen and testosterone levels in the adult male rat, *Acta Endocrinol. (Copenhagen),* 80, 583, 1975.

55. **Damber, J. E. and Bergh, A.,** Decreased testicular response to acute LH-stimulation and increased intratesticular concentration of oestradiol-17β in the abdominal testes in cryptorchid rats, *Acta Endocrinol.,* 95, 416, 1980.

56. **Mulder, E., van Beurden-Lamers, W. M. O., De Boer, W., Brinkman, A. O., and van der Molen, H. J.,** Testicular estradiol receptors in the rats, in *Hormone Binding and Target Cell Activation in the Testis,* Dufau, A. R. and Means, A. R., Eds., Plenum Press, New York, 1974, 343.

57. **Bartke, A., Williams, K. I. H., and Dalterio, S.,** Effects of estrogens on testicular testosterone production *in vitro, Biol. Reprod.,* 17, 645, 1977.

58. **Saez, S. M., Haour, F., Loras, B., Sanches, P., and Cathiard, A. M.,** Oestrogen induced Leydig cell refractoriness to gonadotropin stimulation, *Acta Endocrinol. (Copenhagen),* 89, 379, 1978.

59. **Murono, E. R. and Payne, A. H.,** Distinct testicular 17-ketosteroid reductases, one in the interstitial tissue and one in the seminiferous tubules, *Biochem. Biophys. Acta,* 450, 89, 1976.

60. **Dorrington, J. H. and Armstrong, D. T.,** Follicle-stimulating hormone stimulates estradiol-17β synthesis in cultured Sertoli cells, *Proc. Natl. Acad. Sci. U.S.A.,* 72, 2677, 1975.

61. **Payne, A. H., Kelch, R. P., Musich, S. S., and Halpern, M. E.,** Intratesticular site of aromatization in the human, *J. Clin. Endocrinol. Metab.,* 42, 1081, 1976.

62. **Canick, J. A., Makris, A., Gunsalus, G. L., and Ryan, K. J.,** Testicular aromatization in immature rats: localization and stimulation after gonadotropin administration *in vivo, Endocrinology,* 104, 285, 1979.

63. **Abney, T. O., Grier, H., and Mahesh, V. B.,** Estradiol binding capacity in the cryptorchid rat testis, *Endocrinology,* 101, 975, 1977.

64. **Keel, B. A. and Abney, T. O.,** Influence of bilateral cryptorchidism in the mature rat: alterations in testicular function and serum hormone levels, *Endocrinology,* 107, 1226, 1980.

65. **Keel, B. A. and Abney, T. O.,** Alterations of testicular function in the unilaterally cryptorchid rat, *Proc. Soc. Exp. Biol. Med.,* 166, 489, 1980.

66. **Carter, A. L., Abney, T. O., Braver, H., and Chuang, A. H.,** Localization of γ-butyrobetaine hydroxylase in the rat testis, *Biol. Reprod.,* 37, 68, 1987.

67. **Wisner, J. R. and Gomes, W. R.,** Influence of experimental cryptorchidism on cholesterol side-chain cleavage enzyme and Δ⁵-3β-hydroxysteroid dehydrogenase activities in rat testes, *Steroids,* 31, 189, 1978.

68. **Kormano, M., Harkoner, M., and Kontinen, E.,** Effect of experimental cryptorchidism on the histochemically demonstrable dehydrogenases of the rat testis, *Endocrinology,* 74, 44, 1964.

69. **Christensen, A. K. and Mason, N. R.,** Comparative ability of seminiferous tubules and interstitial tissue of rat testes to synthesize androgens from progesterone-4-¹⁴C *in vitro, Endocrinology,* 76, 646, 1965.

70. **vanDemark, N. L. and Free, M. F.,** Temperature effects, in *The Testis,* Vol. 3, Johnson, A. D., Gomes, W. R., and vanDemark, N. L., Eds., Academic Press, New York, 1970, 233.

71. **Clegg, E. J.,** Studies on artificial cryptorchidism: compensatory changes in the scrotal testis of unilaterally cryptorchid rats, *J. Endocrinol.,* 33, 259, 1965.

72. **Hellbach, G.,** Histochemistrische Untersuchungen an Testes Von Ratten mit hereditar bedingter unilateraler Descensstorungen, Inaugural dissertation, Frankfort am Main, 1970.

73. **Llaurado, J. G. and Dominquez, O. V.,** Effects of cryptorchidism on testicular enzymes involved in androgen biosynthesis, *Endocrinology,* 72, 292, 1963.

74. **Mori, H. and Christensen, A. K.,** Morphometric analysis of Leydig cells in the normal rat testis, *J. Cell Biol.,* 84, 340, 1980.

75. **Payne, A. H., Downing, J. R., and Wong, K. -L.,** Luteinizing hormone receptors and testosterone synthesis in two distinct populations of Leydig cells, *Endocrinology,* 106, 1424, 1980.

76. **Payne, A. H., Wong, K. -L., and Vega, M. M.,** Differential effects of single and repeated administrations of gonadotropins on luteinizing hormone receptors and testosterone synthesis in two populations of Leydig cells, *J. Biol. Chem.,* 255, 7118, 1980.

77. **O'Shaughnessy, P. J., Wong, K. -L., and Payne, A. H.,** Differential steroidogenic enzyme activities in different populations of rat Leydig cells, *Endocrinology,* 109, 1061, 1980.

78. **Georgiou, M. and Payne, A. H.,** 25-Hydroxycholesterol-supported and 8-bromoadenosine 3',5'-monophosphate-stimulated testosterone production by primary cultures of two populations of rat Leydig cells, *Endocrinology,* 117, 1184, 1985.

Chapter 7

CHANGES IN SERTOLI CELL STRUCTURE AND FUNCTION

David M. de Kretser and Gail P. Risbridger

TABLE OF CONTENTS

I. INTRODUCTION

The past decade has witnessed a dramatic increase in our knowledge of the structure and function of the Sertoli cell (for reviews, see References 1 and 2). The pioneering ultrastructural studies established that each Sertoli cell is a distinct cellular entity and not a syncytium. However, subsequent studies have identified that specialized inter-Sertoli cell junctions exist which may facilitate cell-to-cell communication as well as forming the structural basis for the blood-testis barrier.[1,3] The radial orientation of the Sertoli places it in a unique position to influence the environment of a number of different germ cell types since all germ cells, other than spermatogonia, are surrounded by processes of Sertoli cells. This dependence is heightened by the inter-Sertoli cell junctions which prevent intercellular transport of substances into the luminal region of the seminiferous epithelium. Thus, the centrally placed germ cells depend on the Sertoli cells for transport of nutrient materials.

Recent studies have also shown that germ cells utilize lactate as a preferred substrate but are unable to produce this substance.[4,5] They are dependent on the Sertoli cells which metabolize glucose to lactate under the control of follicle-stimulating hormone (FSH).[5-7] Numerous studies have demonstrated that the relationship between Sertoli cells and germ cells is not a one-way phenomenon since the various metabolic functions of the Sertoli cell alter during the stages of the seminiferous cycle (see References 8 and 9). These data suggest that the germ cells in some way modify Sertoli cell activity over a range of functions. Of these numerous functions, those that have been extensively studied are fluid production, androgen-binding protein (ABP) secretion and inhibin secretion in normal rats as well as following the induction of cryptorchidism.[10-13]

The effects of cryptorchidism on these parameters are discussed later in this chapter.

II. ONSET OF CRYPTORCHIDISM

It is worth emphasizing that the time of induction of cryptorchidism may have a significant influence on the changes, not only in spermatogenesis, but also on Sertoli and Leydig cell function. It is well recognized that the longer the cryptorchid state is allowed to persist in congenitally occurring cryptorchidism in man, the more significant the degree of germ cell degeneration.[14]

It attempts to use the rat as a model for human cryptorchidism, a number of investigators have induced cryptorchidism in the neonatal period by cutting the gubernaculum in newborn rats.[15] In numerous other studies, the effect of cryptorchidism has been evaluated in adult rats by surgically relocating the testes into the abdominal cavity and ligating the inguinal canal.[12,16] The important difference between the two induced states derives from the activity of the seminiferous epithelium since in the neonatal period spermatogenesis has barely commenced whereas, in the adult, spermatogenesis is fully developed.

III. CHANGES IN SERTOLI CELL STRUCTURE

The most extensive studies on the changes in Sertoli cell structure associated with the cryptorchidism have been performed in the rat. Neonatal cryptorchidism induced by cutting the gubernaculum results in distinguishable changes in the Sertoli cell at day 16 and in the germ cell complement by 20 d of age.[17] The germ cell changes consist principally of an increase in the number of degenerating germ cells. However, the earliest change consists of an increase in the lipid content of Sertoli cells at day 16.

Subsequently increased vacuolization of Sertoli cells was noted which consisted of two types; the first type resulted from the dilatation of cisternae of smooth endoplasmic reticulum whereas the second specifically involves a dilation of the intercellular space at the sites of

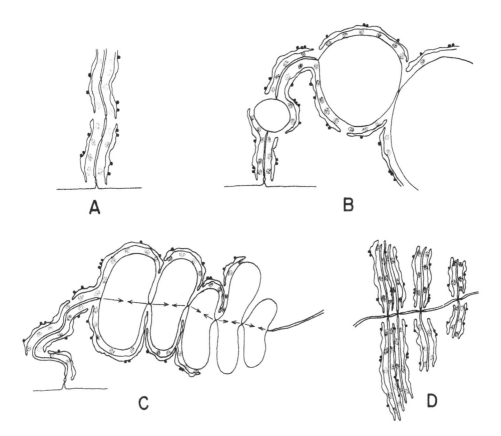

FIGURE 1. Diagrammatic representation of a proposed relationship between the appearance of vacuoles and complex membranous bodies associated with inter-Sertoli cell tight junctions. The hypothesis is based upon observations of the Sertoli cells as cryptorchidism persisted. (A) An inter-Sertoli cell junctional complex within a normal testis. The intercellular space between adjacent Sertoli cells is frequently fused at intervals forming tight junctions. Cisternae of endoplasmic reticulum are separated from the cell surface by hexagonal groups of filaments. (B) After 7 d of cryptorchidism, the intercellular junctions expand between the sites of plasma membrane fusion, giving rise to multiple sites of dilation along the pathway of each junctional complex. The subsurface cisternae expand with the dilated intercellular space, thus usually encompassing each vacuole. (C) With the prompt depletion of germ cells in the sustained cryptorchid state, the Sertoli cells collapse and become compacted. The vacuoles probably undergo compression forces which produce distortion and they behave like a "concertina" mechanism, being squeezed along the pathway of the junctional complex. (D) After 4 weeks of cryptorchidism, the vacuoles are compressed into thin membrane-bound saccules, aggregated in parallel where they form alternate layers with their accompanying cisternae and bundles of filaments. (From Kerr, J. B., Rich, K. A., and de Kretser, D. M., *Biol. Reprod.*, 21, 823, 1979. With permission.)

the inter-Sertoli cell junctions (see Figure 1). Despite these changes in the inter-Sertoli cell junctional complexes, the function of the blood-testis barrier appeared to be intact.[17] It seems likely that the increased lipid in Sertoli cells is not the result of phagocytosis of degenerating germ cells since, when tests without germ cells are made cryptorchid, a similar lipid accumulation occurs.[18] Analysis of the lipid showed an increase in cholesterol and cholesterol esters.[19]

In the adult model, the early changes in Sertoli cell structure are similar to those seen in neonatally induced cryptorchidism and consist of increased numbers of lipid inclusions and dilatations of smooth endoplasmic reticulum.[12] There is also evidence of increased phagocytosis of germ cells. The dilatations of the intercellular space that forms part of the inter-Sertoli cell junctions are distinct and subsequently evolve to produce an unusual structure (Figure 1). The dilatations seem to occur between points at which the Sertoli cell membranes form tight junctions thus forming a chain of dilatations along the length of the inter-Sertoli cell junction.[12] These dilatations subsequently collapse as a result of a "concertina" type of mechanism (Figure 1).

These complexes eventually disappear from the long-term cryptorchid testis. In the latter, there is also an increase in complexity of the interdigitations of Sertoli cell processes in the absence of germ cells. It seems likely that the unusual changes in the inter-Sertoli cell junctions shortly after the induction of cryptorchidism may be the mechanism by which shrinkage in the height of the seminiferous epithelium occurs. This view is made more likely by the observation of similar structural changes in other states wherein there is a rapid loss of germ cells from the epithelium.[20] Long-term cryptorchidism in the rat also results in marked nuclear pleomorphism.

IV. CHANGES IN SERTOLI CELL FUNCTION

As discussed earlier, the Sertoli cell has been credited with an expansive and impressive array of functions in the testis, ranging from the regulation of the maturation of the germ cells, to the production of seminiferous tubule fluid and numerous proteins. Of these it is the production of seminiferous tubule fluid, ABP secretion, and inhibin production that have been thoroughly studied after the induction of cryptorchidism.

V. SEMINIFEROUS TUBULE FLUID PRODUCTION

Seminiferous tubule fluid is transported from the tubule through the rete testis and efferent ducts to the caput epididymis. The major source of fluid is considered to be the Sertoli cell of the tubule rather than the rete testis.[21] The fluid is believed to provide a means of transporting (1) messages from the germ cells to Sertoli cells or vice versa, (2) secretory products from the Sertoli cells, e.g., proteins and hormones to the tubule lumen, and (3) spermatozoa from the tubule lumen to the epididymis. The production of seminiferous tubule fluid requires the development of the blood-testis barrier and the formation of the seminiferous tubule lumen providing a unique microenvironment into which the fluid may be released. Fluid production begins at approximately 20 d of age in the rat[22] and its composition differs from that of plasma.[23] Notably, the potassium concentration is higher, but total protein concentration is much larger in tubule fluid compared to plasma and the composition of the proteins is very different in the two biological fluids (see Reference 23).

Rat seminiferous tubule fluid secretion has been measured as the difference in weights of testes after ligation of the efferent ducts of one side for a period of 16 h. Using this technique, Setchell[23] suggested that fluid production was not under the control of pituitary gonadotrophins based on the observation that seminiferous tubule fluid secretion was not altered for up to 24 h after hypophysectomy of adult rats. However, more recent studies have challenged this view since Jegou and colleagues[24] reported that 3 d after hypophysectomy there is a significant decrease in tubule fluid secretion in the absence of any alteration in testis weight. The latter view has been supported by the results of additional studies.[25]

The induction of cryptorchidism to adult male rats results in the disruption and degeneration of the seminiferous epithelium and an increase in serum gonadotropin levels. The subsequent decline in testis weight is undoubtedly due to a loss of germ cells from the epithelium, but the production of seminiferous tubular fluid also contributes to this decrease. Jegou and colleagues[10] reported a rapid decline within 2 d after surgical induction of cryptorchidism prior to a significant decrease in testis weight (Figure 2). Fluid production continued to fall with extended duration of cryptorchidism, confirming previous observations in both rat and mouse[11,23,26] and indicating an impaired ability of the Sertoli cell to produce fluid. There is no indication as to whether or not the ionic composition of the fluid changes after the

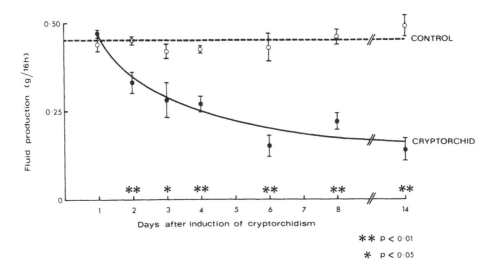

ACUTE EFFECTS OF CRYPTORCHIDISM
ON THE PRODUCTION RATE OF TUBULE FLUID

FIGURE 2. The effect of bilateral cryptorchidism on the accumulation of tubule fluid following efferent duct ligation 16 h previously. Each point is the mean ± SEM (n = 5). (From Jegou, B., Risbridger, G. P., and de Kretser, D. M., *J. Androl.*, 4, 88, 1983. With permission.)

induction of cryptorchidism, although presumably there is an alteration in the concentration of the proteins secreted by the Sertoli cell into the tubule fluid (see below).

While these observations of the effects of surgically induced cryptorchidism in sexually mature rats clearly demonstrate a reduction in tubule fluid production, congenital cryptorchidism is a condition which occurs at birth prior to the establishment of adult Sertoli cell function and spermatogenesis. Therefore, using the technique of cutting the gubernaculum in the newborn rat which results in cryptorchidism, Bergh et al.[15] showed that fluid production increased at 20 d of age.[27] This contrasts with the effects of experimental cryptorchidism induced in the adult male rat[10] and also when cryptorchidism is induced in immature (14-d old) rats.[28] The significance of these differences is unknown.

VI. ANDROGEN-BINDING PROTEIN

Androgen-binding protein is a specific and well-defined product of the Sertoli cell.[29,30] The precise physiological role of ABP is unclear, but it has been suggested that it acts as a carrier of androgens within the Sertoli cell itself, or from the testis to the epididymis.[2] ABP produced by the Sertoli cell is secreted with seminiferous tubule fluid into the lumen and is transported to the duct system of the epididymis where it is taken up by the epithelial cells of the proximal caput region, or secreted into seminal fluid at ejaculation. ABP is also released from the basal surface of the Sertoli cell, is present in testicular fluid, and can be detected in serum or plasma. Thus, the secretion of ABP from the Sertoli cells is bidirectional, although the greater proportion of ABP is released at the luminal aspect of the Sertoli cell. The production of ABP by the Sertoli cell ceases after hypophysectomy but can be restored after treatment with pituitary hormones (LH and FSH).[24,31,32]

Following the experimental induction of cryptorchidism in adult animals, Vernon et al.[33] and Danzo et al.[34] showed a reduction in ABP levels in the rat testis and rabbit epididymis,

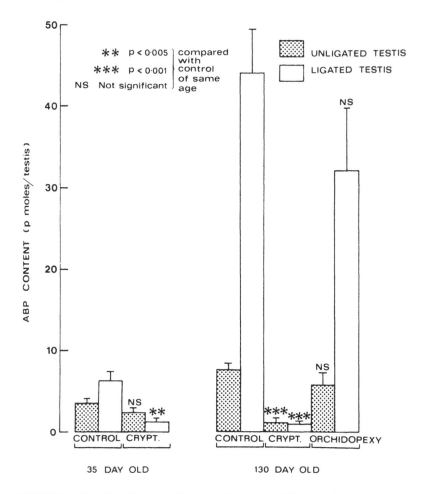

FIGURE 3. The effect of cryptorchidism and subsequent orchidopexy in immature rats on the ABP content and accumulation following unilateral efferent duct ligation 16 h previously. Volumes represent mean + SEM (n = 5). (From Jegou, B., Peake, R. A., Irby, D. C., and de Kretser, D. M., *Biol. Reprod.*, 30, 179, 1984. With permission.)

respectively. This evidence of decreased secretory activity of the Sertoli cell has subsequently been confirmed by a number of other authors in different species.[10-12] Additionally, the experimental induction of cryptorchidism in immature rats results in a reduction (Figure 3) of the testicular ABP content.[28] Finally, in contrast to seminiferous tubule production, ABP levels in the rat made cryptorchid at birth show the same decline indicating an impairment of ABP production by the Sertoli cell.[27] Bergh et al.[27] suggest that the effects of cryptorchidism on Sertoli cell function was more specific than previously suspected. Some of the FSH-stimulated Sertoli cell functions, namely the secretion of ABP, are reduced in cryptorchid testis at an early age when the testes are still descending, but the FSH-dependent tubule fluid production appears to be affected at a later age of development.

The rapid and consistent effects of cryptorchidism on the total content of ABP in testis or epididymal cytosols indicates an overall impairment of the Sertoli cells to produce ABP. The precise manifestations of that impairment remain to be determined. In this context it is possible that the release of ABP from the Sertoli cell may be altered so that a greater proportion of ABP is released at the basal rather than the apical surface of the Sertoli cell thus altering the balance of the bidirectional release of ABP, as suggested by Bardin et al.[35] Nevertheless, the total content of ABP in the testis or epididymis declines after cryptorchidism and reduced capacity of the cryptorchid Sertoli cells to produce ABP *in vitro* is entirely consistent with these observations.[36]

EFFECT OF BILATERAL CRYPTORCHIDISM

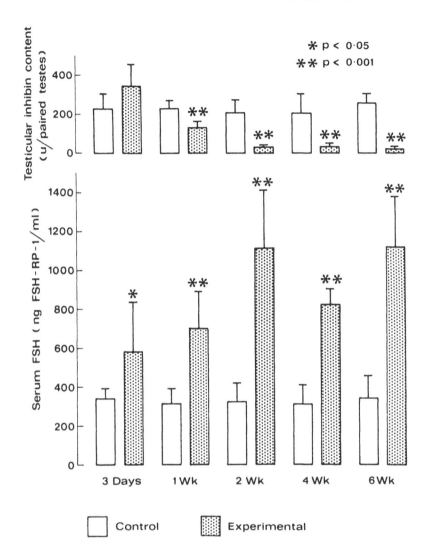

FIGURE 4. Changes in testicular inhibit in content and serum FSH in Sham operated and bilaterally cryptorchid rats at different periods after operation (mean + SD). (From Au, C. L., Robertson, D. M., and de Kretser, D. M., *Endocrinology*, 112, 239, 1983. With permission.)

VII. INHIBIN PRODUCTION

Recent studies have demonstrated that inhibin is a glycoprotein hormone composed of two subunits and is secreted in two forms with molecular weights of 58 and 32 kDa.[37,39] Bioassay measurements indicate that inhibin is secreted by the Sertoli cell and is regulated by FSH.[40,41] More recently, radioimmunoassay measurements have confirmed that inhibin is produced by cultured Sertoli cells and is regulated by FSH.[42]

The induction of experimental cryptorchidism in adult male rats significantly reduced inhibin levels in the testis within 1 week, reaching 10% of the levels (Figure 4) in normal animals by 6 weeks.[13] The accumulation of inhibin measured after efferent duct ligation for 24 h also shows that there is a decline in the production (i.e., synthesis and secretion) of inhibin and that this occurs prior to a decline in the inhibin content of the testis.[43] The reduction in inhibin content in the testis is due to a decrease in inhibin present in the tubules and/or the interstitium.[43] Again, it is not known whether the bidirectional release of inhibin from the Sertoli cells is altered but clearly the total production of inhibin is reduced. These studies are entirely consistent with *in vitro* data demonstrating a progressive decline in the capacity of Sertoli cells isolated from cryptorchid rats testis to synthesize inhibin *in vitro*.[41,44]

The decline in capacity of Sertoli cells to secrete ABP or inhibin after cryptorchidism is inversely correlated with serum concentrations of FSH (and to a lesser extent LH).[10,13] The rise in FSH is probably due to loss of feedback control of the pituitary by inhibin, nevertheless, this provides circumstantial evidence linking impaired Sertoli cell function with elevated levels of FSH in serum.

VIII. SERTOLI CELL SECRETION OF POTENTIAL REGULATORS OF LEYDIG CELLS

Despite the aforementioned observations, Firlitt and Davis[45] and Nagy[46] have reported an increase in the uptake of ^{3}H-leucine by cryptorchid Sertoli cells *in vitro* and *in vivo*. These observations were supported by Rommerts et al.[47] who demonstrated an increased secretion of labeled proteins when Sertoli cells were incubated at 37°C (rather than 32°C), i.e., the temperature to which the crytorchid testis is exposed. Therefore, it would not be surprising to observe a stimulatory effect of cryptorchidism on other Sertoli cell products. One such example is the effect of cryptorchidism on estradiol secretion. Testosterone produced by the Leydig cells may be converted to estradiol in the immature testis by the action of the aromatase enzyme. The induction of bilateral cryptorchidism increases estradiol levels in serum[48] and in the testis[49] and the capacity of the cryptorchid testis to produce estradiol *in vitro* is significantly increased.[50] However, an earlier report by Hall and Gomes[51] indicates that estradiol levels were only transiently elevated after experimental cryptorchidism and then declined. The reason for these discrepant data is unclear.

Estradiol was known to have a direct inhibitory effect on steroidogenesis[52] and it was postulated that estradiol produced by the Sertoli cells in the tubules could act locally to regulate Leydig cell steroidogenesis. This putative local or paracrine action of estrogens in the testis was not supported by the fact that after the induction of cryptorchidism in the rat, the function of the Leydig cells appeared to be stimulated further rather than inhibited.[53] Furthermore, the ability of rat Sertoli cells to aromatize testosterone disappeared at 18 to 20 d of age and the Leydig cell was the principal site of production of estradiol.[54,55]

There is considerable interest in the identification of local factors emanating from the seminiferous tubules which can regulate Leydig cell steroidogenesis. Both inhibitory and stimulating activities have been identified in cultures of tubules or Sertoli cells or in testicular interstitial fluid. However, relatively few examinations of the effects of cryptorchidism on these activities have been undertaken. Syed and colleagues[56] have reported the presence of activity in spent media from incubated seminiferous tubules which inhibits testosterone production by Leydig cells *in vitro*. Upon the induction of cryptorchidism, one would predict a decrease in the inhibitory activity in order to account for the observed hyperresponsiveness of Leydig cells. Indeed, this group showed a gradual disappearance in the inhibitor activity after the induction of cryptorchidism and the emergence of a stimulatory activity.[57] The authors concluded that the seminiferous tubules of the cryptorchid rat are the source of a heat-labile, trypsin-resistant factor of MW 5000—10,000 daltons. In the normal adult rat a factor capable of stimulating Leydig cell steroidogenesis has been reported to be present in testicular interstitial fluid[58] (see Chapter 8) which again is consistent with the hypothesis that more of a local stimulatory factor is produced after damage to the seminiferous epithelium by the induction of cryptorchidism resulting in stimulation of Leydig cells. Further work is

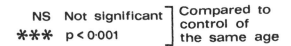

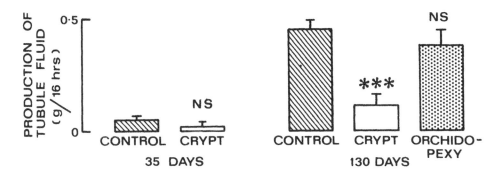

FIGURE 5. The effect of cryptorchidism and subsequent orchidopexy in immature rats on the production of tubule fluid at 35 and 130 d of age (mean + SEM, n = 5). (From Jegou, B., Peake, R. A., Irby, D. C., and de Kretser, D. M., *Biol. Reprod.*, 30, 179, 1984. With permission.)

required to isolate the factor or factors produced by the seminiferous tubules or which are present in testicular interstitial fluid which affect Leydig cell steroidogenesis.

IX. CAN RECOVERY OCCUR AFTER ORCHIDOPEXY?

There is considerable confusion concerning the degree of recovery that can occur following reversal of experimental cryptorchidism by orchidopexy. Some investigators have claimed excellent restoration of testicular function while others have had disappointing results.[16,59,60] Some of this confusion is the result of numerous regimes that have been employed with variations occurring in the age of induction of cryptorchidism, the duration of the cryptorchid state, and the surgical techniques involved. To simplify this section we have divided this discussion into (1) reversal of cryptorchidism induced in sexually immature animals and (2) reversal of cryptorchidism induced in sexually mature animals.

A. Reversal of Cryptorchidism Induced in Sexually Immature Animals

In general, there is good recovery of spermatogenesis if the cryptorchid state is of short duration and is carefully corrected.[28,61] It is only in recent times that effects on Sertoli and Leydig cell function have been monitored. In rats made cryptorchid at day 14 and reversed at day 35, the alterations in Leydig cell and Sertoli cell function (Figures 3 to 5) noted at day 35 are completely reversed.[8,61] This reversal links the changes in Leydig cell function closely to events occurring within the seminiferous tubules, a view discussed further in the following section.

B. Reversal of Cryptorchidism Induced in Sexually Mature Animals

There are claims of complete recovery of the spermatogenic function of testis in rats with a long duration of cryptorchidism.[16] However, several recent studies have been unable to document these excellent results.[59,60] In our own studies we observed that if the cryptorchid state was allowed to persist for more than 2 weeks, recovery of spermatogenesis was poor as was the impairment of Sertoli cell function.[60] However, if the duration was 10 d, some rats recovered spermatogenic function whereas in others there was a continuing impairment of spermatogenic and Sertoli cell function. If the rats were divided according to whether

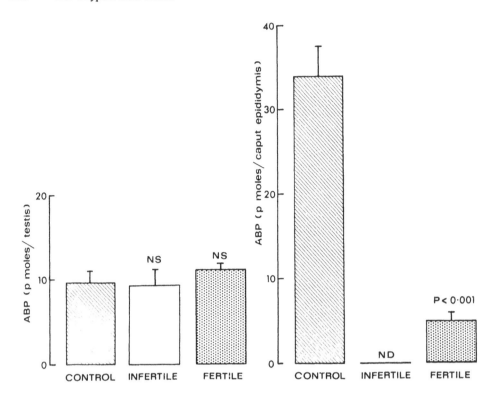

FIGURE 6.   ABP content in the testis and epididymis of control rats that were fertile or infertile 6 months after orchidopexy which was preceeded by a 10-d period of cryptorchidism (mean + SEM, n = 5; ND, non-detectable).

recovery occurred or failed, there were corresponding changes in Sertoli cell and Leydig cell function. In those rats which recovered, Sertoli cell function improved and the hyperresponsiveness of the Leydig cell also returned to normal (Figures 6 and 7). In those with poor spermatogenic recovery, Sertoli cell function was impaired and Leydig cell hyperresponsiveness persisted. This relationship provides further evidence that the Leydig cells are influenced by the function of the seminiferous tubules (see References 9, 62, and 63). Similar correlations between hyperresponsive Leydig cells and impaired seminiferous tubule function have been noted in numerous other models of spermatogenic disruption.[61-65] The mechanisms involved remain unknown but inhibitors and stimulators of Leydig cell function have been reported in media from cultures of seminiferous tubules and Sertoli cells.[56,57,66,67] Further resolution of this problem requires the purification and in-depth characterization of the substances responsible for these activities.

X. IS THERE A PARALLEL TO HUMAN CRYPTORCHIDISM?

Results from studies of experimental cryptorchidism confirm the relationship that the longer the duration of cryptorchidism, the more severe the spermatogenic defect.[14] However, it should be noted that in many instances reversal of cryptorchidism in boys has not restored spermatogenesis and the results raise the question of whether some basic defect in the testis is responsible for both the failure of descent and the persisting spermatogenic defect (see Reference 68 for review). This is particularly pertinent to those males with unilateral testicular maldescent who are infertile due to oligospermia.

Unfortunately, tests of Sertoli cell function are not currently available in man although the degree of elevation of FSH levels in serum may provide circumstantial evidence of a

INCREMENTAL RISE OF TESTOSTERONE

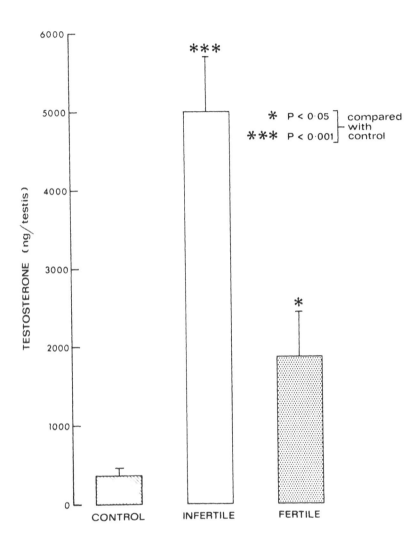

FIGURE 7.   Incremental rise in the production of testosterone in response to hCG stimulation *in vitro* in control rats and those that were fertile or infertile 6 months after orchidopexy which was preceded by a 10-d period of cryptorchidism, (mean + SEM, n = 5).

decline in inhibin production. The recent purification of inhibin[37] and the cloning of its genes[69,70] have allowed the development of radioimmunoassays for this hormone in man.[71] The latter will allow exploration of whether circulating inhibin levels can be used as a marker of Sertoli cell function.

Altered Leydig cell function is seen in men with severe testicular damage resulting from persistent cryptorchidism or failed orchidopexy. There is evidence of decreased or normal testosterone and elevated LH levels suggesting Leydig cell failure, namely, higher than normal LH levels being required to maintain normal testosterone levels.[72,73] These changes are not restricted to cryptorchidism but may result from other types of testicular damage. Whether human Leydig cells are also hyperresponsive *in vitro* and show a decline in LH receptors as seen in the cryptorchid rat testis must await further data. However, there is no doubt that persisting spermatogenic failure is associated with changes in Leydig cell function in man.

REFERENCES

1. **Fawcett, D. W.,** Ultrastructure and function of the Sertoli cell, in *Handbook of Physiology,* Greep, R. O. and Hamilton, D. W., Eds., Williams & Wilkins, Baltimore, 1975, 21.
2. **Ritzen, E. M., Hansson, V., and French, F. S.,** The Sertoli cell, in *The Testis,* Burger, H. G. and de Kretser, D. M., Eds., Raven Press, New York, 1981, 171.
3. **Dym, M. and Fawcett, D. W.,** The blood-testis barrier in the rat and the physiological compartmentation of the seminiferous epithelium, *Biol. Reprod.,* 3, 308, 1970.
4. **Jutte, N. H. P. M., Grootegoed, J. A., Rommerts, F. F. G., and van der Molen, H. J.,** Exogenous lactate is essential for metabolic activity in isolated rat spermatocytes and spermatids, *J. Reprod. Fertil.,* 62, 399, 1981.
5. **Mita, M., Price, J. M., and Hall, P. F.,** Stimulation by FSH of synthesis of lactate by Sertoli cells from rat testis, *Endocrinology,* 110, 1535, 1982.
6. **Jutte, N. H. P. M., Jansen, R., Grootegoed, A. J., Rommerts, F. F. G., Clausen, O. P. F., and van der Molen, H. J.,** Regulation of survival of rat pachytene spermatocytes by lactate supply from Sertoli cells, *J. Reprod. Fertil.,* 65, 431, 1982.
7. **Jutte, N. H. P. M., Jansen, R., Grootegoed, J. A., Rommerts, F. F. G. and van der Molen, H. J.,** FSH stimulation of the production of pyruvate and lactate by rat Sertoli cells may be involved in hormonal regulation of spermatogenesis, *J. Reprod. Fertil.,* 68, 219, 1983.
8. **Parvinen, M.,** Regulation of the seminiferous epithelium, *Endocr. Rev.,* 3, 404, 1982.
9. **Sharpe, R. M.,** Paracrine control of the testis, *Clin. Endocrinol. Metab.,* 15, 185, 1986.
10. **Jegou, B., Risbridger, G. P., and de Kretser, D. M.,** Effects of experimental cryptorchidism on testicular function in adult rats, *J. Androl.,* 4, 88, 1983.
11. **Hagenas, L. and Ritzen, E. M.,** Impaired Sertoli cell function in experimental cryptorchidism, *Mol. Cell. Endocrinol.,* 4, 25, 1976.
12. **Kerr, J. B., Rich, K. A., and de Kretser, D. M.,** Effects of experimental cryptorchidism on the ultrastructure and function of the Sertoli cell and peritubular tissue of the rat testis, *Biol. Reprod.,* 21, 823, 1979.
13. **Au, C. L., Robertson, D. M., and de Kretser, D. M.,** In vitro bioassay of inhibin in testes of normal and cryptorchid rats, *Endocrinology,* 112, 239, 1983.
14. **Mancini, R. E., Rosemberg, E., Cullen, M., Lavieri, J. C., Vilar, O., Bergada, C., and Andrada, J. A.,** Cryptorchid and scrotal human testes. I. Cytological cytochemical and quantitative studies, *J. Clin. Endocrinol. Metab.,* 25, 927, 1965.
15. **Bergh, A., Helander, H. F., and Wahlquist, L.,** Studies on factors governing testicular descent in the rat — particularly the role of gubernaculum testis, *Int. J. Androl.,* 1, 342, 1978.
16. **Nelson, W. O.,** Mammalian spermatogenesis: effect of experimental cryptorchidism in the rat and nondescent of the testis in man, *Rec. Prog. Horm. Res.,* 6, 29, 1951.
17. **Bergh, A.,** Early morphological changes in the abdominal testes in immature unilaterally cryptorchid rats, *Int. J. Androl.,* 6, 73, 1983.
18. **Bergh, A.,** Morphological signs of a direct effect of experimental cryptorchidism on the Sertoli cells in rats irradiated as fetuses, *Biol. Reprod.,* 24, 145, 1981.
19. **Fleger, J. L., Bishop, J. P., Gomey, W. R. and van Demark, N. L.,** Testicular lipids. I. Effect of unilateral cryptorchidism on lipid classes, *J. Reprod. Fertil.,* 15, 1, 1968.
20. **de Kretser, D. M. and Kerr, J. B.,** The cytology of the testis, in *The Physiology of Reproduction,* Knobil, E. and Neill, J. D., Eds., Raven Press, New York, in press.
21. **Setchell, B. P.,** Do Sertoli cells secrete fluid into the seminiferous tubules?, *J. Reprod. Fertil.,* 19, 391, 1969.
22. **Jegou, B., Le Gac, F., and de Kretser, D. M.,** Seminiferous tubule fluid and interstitial fluid production. I. Effects of age and hormonal regulators in immature rats, *Biol. Reprod.,* 27, 590, 1982.
23. **Setchell, B. P.,** The secretion of fluid by the testis of rats, ram and goats with some observations on the effect of age, cryptorchidism and hypophysectomy, *J. Reprod. Fertil.,* 23, 79, 1970.
24. **Jegou, B., Le Gac, F., Irby, D., and de Kretser, D. M.,** Studies on seminiferous tubule fluid production in the adult rat: effect of hypophysectomy and treatment with FSH, LH and testosterone, *Int. J. Androl.,* 6, 249, 1983.
25. **Au, C. L., Robertson, D. M., and de Kretser, D. M.,** Effects of hypophysectomy and subsequent FSH and testosterone treatment on inhibin production by adult rat testes, *J. Endocrinol.,* 105, 1, 1985.
26. **Barrack, B. M.,** Transport of spermatozoa from seminiferous tubules to epididymis in the mouse: a histological and quantitative study, *J. Reprod. Fertil.,* 16, 35, 1968.
27. **Bergh, A., Damber, J. E., and Ritzen, M.,** Early signs of Sertoli and Leydig cell dysfunction in the abdominal testes of immature unilaterally cryptorchid rats, *Int. J. Androl.,* 7, 398, 1984.
28. **Jegou, B., Peake, R. A., Irby, D. C., and de Kretser, D. M.,** Effects of the induction of experimental cryptorchidism and subsequent orchidopexy on testicular function in immature rats, *Biol. Reprod.,* 30, 179, 1984.

29. **Ritzen, E. M., Dobbins, M. C., Tindall, D. J., French, F. S., and Nayfeh, S. N.,** Characterization of androgen-binding protein (ABP) in rat testis and epididymis, *Steroids*, 21, 593, 1973.

30. **Hagenas, L., Ritzen, E. M., Ploen, L., Hansson, V., French, F. S., and Nayfeh, S. N.,** Sertoli cell origin of testicular androgen binding protein (ABP), *Mol. Cell. Endocrinol.*, 2, 339, 1975.

31. **Hansson, V., Reusch, E., Trugstad, O., Torgersen, O., Ritzen, E. M., and French, F. S.,** FSH stimulation of testicular androgen binding protein, *Nature*, 246, 56, 1973.

32. **Fritz, I. B., Rommerts, F. F. G., Louis, B. G., and Dorrington, J. H.,** Regulation by FSH and cAMP of the formation of ABP in Sertoli cell-enriched cultures, *J. Reprod. Fertil.*, 46, 17, 1976.

33. **Vernon, R. G., Kopec, B., and Fritz, I. B.,** Observations on the binding of androgens by rat testis seminiferous tubules and testis extracts, *Mol. Cell. Endocrinol.*, 1, 167, 1974.

34. **Danzo, B. J., Eller, B. C., and Orgebin-Crist, M. C.,** Studies on the site of origin of the androgen binding protein present in epididymal cytosol from mature intact rabbits, *Steroids*, 24, 107, 1974.

35. **Bardin, C. W., Larreaf Gunsalas, G. L., and Musto, N. A.,** Testicular androgen binding protein in the rat physical & physiological studies, *6th Int. Congr. Endocrinol.*, Abstr. S24, 137, 1980.

36. **Le Gac, F. and de Kretser, D. M.,** Studies on isolated Sertoli cells from normal and cryptorchid testis, *6th Int. Congr. Endocrinol.*, Abstr. 684, 551, 1980.

37. **Robertson, D. M., Foulds, L. M., Leversha, L., Morgan, F. J., Hearn, M. T. W., Burger, H. G., Wettenhall, R. E. H., and de Kretser, D. M.,** Isolation of inhibin from bovine follicular fluid, *Biochem. Biophys. Res. Commun.*, 126, 220, 1985.

38. **Robertson, D. M., de Vos, F. L., Foulds, L. M., McLachlan, R. I., Burger, H. G., Morgan, F. J., Hearn, M. T. W., and de Kretser, D. M.,** Isolation of a 31 kDa form of inhibin from bovine follicular fluid, *Mol. Cell. Endocrinol.*, 44, 271, 1986.

39. **Miyamoto, K., Hasegawa, Y., Fukuda, M., Nomura, M., Igarashi, M., Kangawa, K., and Matsuo, H.,** Isolation of porcine follicular fluid inhibin of 32 K daltons, *Biochem. Biophys. Res. Commun.*, 129, 396, 1985.

40. **Steinberger, A. and Steinberger, E.,** Secretion of an FSH-inhibiting factor by cultured Sertoli cells, *Endocrinology*, 99, 918, 1976.

41. **Le Gac, F. and de Kretser, D. M.,** Inhibin production by Sertoli cell cultures, *Mol. Cell. Endocrinol.*, 28, 487, 1982.

42. **Bisak, T., Vale, W., Vaughan, J., Tucker, E., Chappel, S., and Hsueh, A. J. W.,** Hormonal regulation of inhibin production by cultured Sertoli cells, *Mol. Cell. Endocrinol.*, 49, 211, 1987.

43. **Au, C. L., Robertson, D. M., and de Kretser, D. M.,** An in vivo method for estimating inhibin production by adult rat testes, *J. Reprod. Fertil.*, 71, 259, 1985.

44. **Seethalakshi, L. and Steinberger, A.,** Effect of cryptorchidism and orchidopexy on inhibin secretion by rat Sertoli cells, *J. Androl.*, 4, 131, 1983.

45. **Firlitt, E. F. and Davis, J. R.,** Radioautographic incorporation of L-lysine-3H into protein in cells of the germinal epithelium in cryptorchidism, *J. Reprod. Fertil.*, 11, 125, 1986.

46. **Nagy, F.,** Tritiated leucine incorporation by Sertoli cells in scrotal and cryptorchid rat testis, *Fertil. Steril.*, 24, 805, 1973.

47. **Rommerts, F. F. G., de Jong, F. J., Grootegoed, J. A., and van der Molen, H. J.,** Metabolic changes in testicular cells from rats after long term exposure to 37°C in vivo or in vitro, *J. Endocrinol.*, 85, 471, 1980.

48. **Jones, T. M., Anderson, W., Fang, V. S., Landau, R. L., and Rosenfield, R. L.,** Experimental cryptorchidism in adult male rats: histological and hormonal sequelae, *Anat. Rec.*, 189, 1, 1977.

49. **Damber, J. G. and Bergh, A.,** Decreased testicular response to acute LH-stimulation & increased intra-testicular concentration of oestradiol 17-β in the abdominal testis in cryptorchid rats, *Acta Endocrinol.*, 95, 416, 1980.

50. **de Kretser, D. M., Sharpe, R. M., and Swanston, I. A.,** Alterations in steroidogenesis and human chorionic gonadotrophin binding in the cryptorchid rat testis, *Endocrinology*, 105, 135, 1979.

51. **Hall, P. F. and Gomes, W. R.,** The effect of artificial cryptorchidism on serum oestrogen and testosterone levels in the adult male rat, *Acta Endocrinol.*, 80, 583, 1975.

52. **Hseuh, A. J. W., Dufau, M., and Catt, K. J.,** Direct inhibitory effect of estrogen on Leydig cell function of hypophysectomized rats, *Endocrinology*, 103, 1096, 1978.

53. **Risbridger, G. P., Kerr, J. B., and de Kretser, D. M.,** An evaluation of Leydig cell function and gonadotrophin binding in unilateral and bilateral cryptorchidism. Evidence for local control of Leydig cell function by the seminiferous tubule, *Biol. Reprod.*, 24, 534, 1981.

54. **Pomerantz, D. K.,** Effects of in vivo gonadotrophin treatment on estrogen levels in the testis of the immature rats, *Biol. Reprod.*, 21, 1247, 1979.

55. **Valladares, L. E. and Payne, A. H.,** Induction of testicular aromatization by luteinizing hormone in mature rats, *Endocrinology*, 105, 431, 1979.

56. **Syed, V., Khan, S. A., and Ritzen, E. M.,** Stage-specific inhibition of interstitial cell testosterone secretion by rat seminiferous tubules in vitro, *Mol. Cell. Endocrinol.*, 40, 257, 1985.

57. **Syed, V., Karpe, B., Ploen, L., and Ritzen, E. M.**, Regulation of interstitial cell function by seminiferous tubules in intact and cryptorchid rats, *Int. J. Androl.*, 9, 127, 1986.

58. **Sharpe, R. M., Doogan, D. G., and Cooper, I.**, Intratesticular factors and testosterone secretion: the role of luteinizing hormone in relation to changes during puberty and experimental cryptorchidism, *Endocrinology*, 119, 2089, 1986.

59. **Hayashi, H. and Cedento, A. P.**, Fertilizing capacity of the cryptorchid rat, *J. Reprod. Fertil.*, 59, 79, 1980.

60. **Jegou, B., Laws, A. O., and de Kretser, D. M.**, The effect of cryptorchidism and subsequent orchidopexy on testicular function in adult rats, *J. Reprod. Fertil.*, 69, 137, 1983.

61. **Karpe, B., Ploen, L., Hagenas, L., and Ritzen, E. M.**, Recovery of testicular function after surgical treatment of experimental cryptorchidism in the rat, *Int. J. Androl.*, 4, 145, 1981.

62. **de Kretser, D. M.**, Sertoli cell-Leydig cell interaction in the regulation of testicular function, *Int. J. Androl.*, 5, 11, 1982.

63. **de Kretser, D. M.**, Local regulation of testicular function, *Int. Rev. Cytol.*, in press.

64. **Jegou, B., Laws, A. O., and de Kretser, D. M.**, Changes in testicular function induced by short term exposure of the rat testis to the heat: further evidence for interaction of germ cells, Sertoli cells and Leydig cells, *Int. J. Androl.*, 7, 244, 1984.

65. **Au, C. L., Robertson, D. M., and de Kretser, D. M.**, Changes in testicular inhibin following a single episode of heating of rat testes, *Endocrinology*, in press.

66. **Verhoeven, G. and Cailleau, J.**, A factor in spent media from Sertoli cell-enriched cultures that stimulates steroidogenesis in Leydig cells, *Mol. Cell. Endocrinol.*, 40, 57, 1985.

67. **Benhamed, M., Morera, A. M., and Chauvin, M. A.**, Evidence for a Sertoli cell, FSH-suppressible inhibiting factor(s) of testicular steroidogenic activity, *Biochem. Biophys. Res. Commun.*, 139, 169, 1986.

68. **Sizoneuko, P. C., Schindler, A. M., and Guendet, A.**, Clinical evaluation and management of testicular disorders before puberty, in *The Testis*, Burger, H. and de Kretser, D. M., Eds., Raven Press, New York, 1981, 303.

69. **Mason, A. J., Hayflick, J. S., Ling, N., Esch, F., Ueno, N., Ying, S. Y., Gullemin, R., Niall, H., and Seeburg, P. H.**, Complementary DNA sequences of ovarian follicular fluid inhibin show precursor structure and homology with transforming growth factor B, *Nature*, 318, 659, 1985.

70. **Forage, R. G., Ring, J. M., Brown, R. W., McInerey, B. V., Cobon, G. S., Gregson, R. P., Robertson, D. M., Morgan, F. J., Hearn, M. T. W., Findlay, J. K., Wettenhall, R. E. N., Burger, H. G., and de Kretser, D. M.**, Cloning and sequence analysis of cDNA species coding for the two subunits of inhibin from bovine follicular fluid, *Proc. Nat. Acad. Sci. U.S.A.*, 83, 3091, 1986.

71. **McLachlan, R. I., Robertson, D. M., Burger, H. G., and de Kretser, D. M.**, The radioimmunoassay of bovine follicular fluid inhibin, *Mol. Cell. Endocrinol.*, 46, 175, 1986.

72. **de Kretser, D. M., Burger, H. G., Fortune, D., Hudson, B., Long, A., Paulsen, C. A., and Taft, H. P.**, Hormonal, histological and genetic studies on male infertility, *J. Clin. Endocrinol. Metab.*, 35, 392, 1972.

73. **de Kretser, D. M., Burger, H. G., Hudson, B., and Keogh, E. J.**, The hCG stimulation test in men with testicular disorders, *Clin. Endocrinol.*, 4, 591, 1975.

Chapter 8

SERTOLI-LEYDIG CELL INTERACTIONS IN THE UNILATERALLY CRYPTORCHID TESTIS

Jeffrey B. Kerr and Richard M. Sharpe

TABLE OF CONTENTS

I. INTRODUCTION

It is now accepted that normal testicular function is dependent upon multiple interactions between all of the different cell types in the testis.[1-3] Potentially, one of the most important of these interactions is that between the Sertoli and Leydig cells, because it is the latter that supply the testosterone which acts on the Sertoli cells to drive spermatogenesis. Because of the dependence of spermatogenesis, and hence fertility, on an adequate supply of testosterone by the Leydig cells to the Sertoli cells, it is not surprising that several mechanisms have been shown to exist via which the Sertoli cells can exert paracrine control of the Leydig cells.[1-3] In addition, it is now recognized that the Leydig cells are the source of at least two other hormones, oxytocin and opiates such as β-endorphin,[1] the former of which acts on the peritubular myoid cells[4] and the latter on the Sertoli cells.[5] Multiple feedback signals may, therefore, be generated by the Sertoli cells to control the secretion of one or more of these Leydig cell products.

Experimental cryptorchidism has been used widely because it results in rapid and gross impairment of spermatogenesis and, hence, of Sertoli cell function.[6] In view of the latter changes, alterations in Leydig cell structure and/or function might also be expected, secondary to changes in secretion by the Sertoli cell of the paracrine hormones which exert feedback control of the Leydig cells. In this respect the unilaterally cryptorchid rat[6-9] has been the favored model as it permits evaluation of the relative roles of systemic (i.e., pituitary hormones) and local (i.e., intratesticular paracrine hormones) factors in control of the Leydig cells. If changes are observed in the abdominal but not in the scrotal testis, then it can be concluded that this change is at least partly dependent on local factors.[6] The purpose of the present chapter is to detail these changes and what they mean in terms of Leydig cell numbers, morphology, and function, and how these relate to changes in one of the paracrine factors which may be involved in local control of the Leydig cells. It should be emphasized that there is a fairly extensive literature on Leydig cell changes in the unilaterally cryptorchid rat (see below) and much of the present chapter represents a reevaluation of previous studies in light of the most recent findings, which are presented below.

II. CHANGES IN LEYDIG CELL MORPHOLOGY AND NUMBERS

There is a considerable volume of direct and indirect evidence, from both morphological[6,8,10,11] and functional,[6,7,12-14] studies to show that spermatogenic disruption such as that which occurs in cryptorchidism results in altered Leydig cell function, and these changes are probably induced by local intratesticular factors rather than solely due to circulating gonadotropic hormones. Leydig cell biology after unilateral cryptorchidism has been studied in adult rats[6,7,9,13] and in newborn rats[8,11,14,15] the latter simulating congenitally related cryptorchidism. Both of these approaches produce seminiferous tubule damage, but the reported cytological changes to the Leydig cells are rather different. In rats made unilaterally cryptorchid after birth,[8] Leydig cell size, total volume, and number per abdominal testis after 4 weeks is not different from the same measurements made in the scrotal testis. However, at 100 d after surgery in the same experiment, Leydig cell numbers per abdominal and scrotal testis are the same, yet the abdominal Leydig cells become smaller and thus total Leydig cell volume in abdominal testes is reduced significantly compared to the contralateral scrotal testes. Similar data have been reported by Bergh et al.[16] yet nothing is known about the factors which bring about shrinkage or atrophy of the Leydig cells. The latter report suggested that the smaller abdominal Leydig cells contained less endoplasmic reticulum, and this is believed to reflect the poor steroid secretion *in vivo*[8,16] of these cells. Entirely opposite observations on the morphology of Leydig cells have been described for rats made unilaterally cryptorchid as adults, in which abdominal Leydig cells were hypertrophied compared to the scrotal Leydig cells.[6] Similar data is available from studies of Leydig cells in bilaterally cryptorchid rats[17,18] in which the abdominal Leydig cells were found to be enlarged compared to scrotal Leydig cells in intact rats. When examined by electron microscopy and sterological methods,[18] the abdominal Leydig cells exhibited significant increases in the total volume of organelles in their cytoplasm. The hypertrophy of abdominal Leydig cells following uni- or bilateral lesion of the testis is believed to correlate well with the increased testosterone response to hCG stimulation *in vitro* (see below and References 6 and 7). A third, but less often used, age group selected for experimental cryptorchidism has been the 2-week-old rat in which abdominal Leydig cells of bilaterally cryptorchid testes were reported to enlarge compared to scrotal Leydig cells in age-matched intact rats.[19] Thus, the induction of unilateral cryptorchidism in either newborn or immature/adult rats can induce atrophy or hypertrophy, respectively, of the abdominal Leydig cells. Since no unifying hypothesis has emerged which provides a satisfactory explanation for these apparently paradoxical findings, the effect of unilateral cryptorchidism in adult rats upon Leydig cell cytology has been thoroughly reexamined using contemporary stereological techniques.

III. REINVESTIGATION OF THE RESPONSE OF LEYDIG CELLS TO CRYPTORCHIDISM

Histological and morphometric analyses of the testes were performed in four groups of rats consisting of a control group of intact rats and rats which had been made unilaterally cryptorchid as adults and which were killed in three groups at 1, 2, and 4 weeks after induction of cryptorchidism. The ten rats in each group were killed with ether, blood was collected by cardiac aspiration, and the serum separated and stored at −20°C until assayed for FSH, LH, and testosterone.[20] Testes from three rats in each group were perfusion fixed with a buffered glutaraldehyde-formaldehyde mixture. The testes were decapsulated, their volumes measured, and small blocks of tissue were postfixed in osmium tetroxide, processed, and embedded in epoxy resin using standard methods previously described.[18,21] One-micron sections were stained with toluidine blue and quantitative analysis of total Leydig cell volume and numbers per testis from all animals was performed by light microscopy using methods described earlier.[22,23]

In intact control testes, Leydig cells exhibited the usual features seen in adult rat testes: a distribution around blood vessels or singly or in small clusters in random locations within the interstitial tissue (Figure 1). The morphology of the interstitial tissue and the Leydig cells appeared unchanged in all of the sections examined from the scrotal testes of unilaterally cryptorchid rats. Disruption of spermatogenesis occurred in the abdominal testes, the severity of which increased with the duration of cryptorchidism. The Leydig cells of abdominal testes tended to cluster around the interstitial blood vessels as the degenerating seminiferous tubules contracted in diameter (Figures 2 to 4). No other noteworthy morphological alterations were recorded for the abdominal Leydig cells, since in purely qualitative terms, they appeared neither markedly enlarged nor shrunken in size. By light microscopy, abdominal Leydig cells presented a prominent nucleus and their cytoplasm was often filled with dense granules representing mitochondria. When examined by electron microscopy (Figures 5 and 6), the abdominal Leydig cells showed many more mitochondria than scrotal Leydig cells. Results of morphometric analysis are presented in Table 1.

After 1, 2, and 4 weeks of unilateral cryptorchidism, testicular volume was reduced significantly in abdominal testes to 46, 29 and 21%, respectively, of the volume of the contralateral scrotal testes. Volumetric density of Leydig cells, i.e., that volume proportion of the testis occupied by Leydig cells, ranged from 2.4 to 3.0% in scrotal testes, regardless of whether the testes were from intact or cryptorchid animals. In contrast, the volumetric density of Leydig cells in abdominal testes was increased significantly by two- to fourfold.

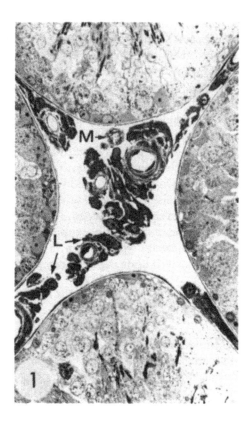

FIGURE 1.   Interstitial tissue of normal adult rat testis
showing basophilic Leydig cells (L) and a macrophage
(M). (Magnification × 380.)

Therefore, in a simple inspection of the stained 1-μm sections of testicular tissues, the impression gained was of relative hyperplasia of the Leydig cells. However, since the volume of abdominal testes was reduced markedly, the conversion of volumetric density data of Leydig cells into total volume of Leydig cells in microliter per testis revealed a completely different picture, in that there was no difference in the absolute volumes of Leydig cells in abdominal or scrotal testes. When total Leydig cell numbers per testis were calculated using data obtained for the size and number of Leydig cell nuclei as described above,[23] no differences were found between the values in abdominal or scrotal testes.

The animals belonging to each of the groups (n = 3) were derived from a larger series in which each group contained ten animals and serum collected from these was examined for the levels of follicle-stimulating hormone (FSH), luteinizing hormone (LH), and testosterone in the peripheral circulation. Serum FSH and LH were increased significantly in unilaterally cryptorchid animals compared to the intact control group, although serum testosterone tended to be somewhat lower (Figure 7). In spite of elevated gonadotropin levels in serum, the morphometric data indicate that the gonadotropins failed to alter the total volume or total numbers of Leydig cells in abdominal vs. scrotal testes. Thus, these findings differ from previous reports of Leydig cell atrophy in abdominal testes of rats, aged 100 d, which had been made unilaterally cryptorchid at birth.[8] The present data are also in contrast to earlier observations of Leydig cell hypertrophy in abdominal testes of 2- or 4-week uni- or bilaterally cryptorchid adult rats,[6,18] or in abdominal testes of adult rats made bilaterally cryptorchid at 2 weeks of age.[19] One possible explanation for these divergent findings is that each set of data was based upon differing methods of assessing Leydig cell size, individual volume, and total numbers per testis, introducing the possibility that the collection

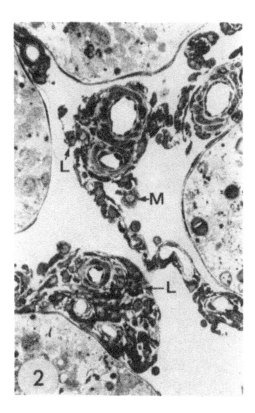

FIGURE 2. Abdominal testis of a 1-week unilaterally cryptorchid rat showing numerous Leydig cells (L). Macrophages (M) also indicated. (Magnification × 380.)

of quantitative data is influenced by the manner in which the data were obtained. For example, the reported atrophy of abdominal Leydig cells in rats made unilaterally cryptorchid at birth[8] was based not upon direct measurements of Leydig cell size in semithin sections, but upon results from two other sets of data, namely the ratio between Leydig cell volumetric density and the numerical density of Leydig cells. In any comparison of these findings from neonatally operated animals and those presented here for adult-operated animals the following points should be considered:

1. The differences in the response of Leydig cell volume in abdominal and scrotal testes is seen in the long-term (100 d-old) neonatally operated rats, but in 4-week-old rats in the same experiment no changes in the measured Leydig cell parameters was noted when abdominal and scrotal Leydig cells were examined. At this time point the present results for adult rats are identical to neonatally operated rats.
2. The Leydig cells of adult unilaterally cryptorchid rats have not been examined after a period of 100 d and it could be that they also undergo atrophy at this time.

The data presented here are not suggestive of Leydig cell hyperplasia or hypertrophy following induction of cryptorchidism, a proposal which has been put forward in the past and which was based upon two observations: (1) ultrastructural evidence of mitotic activity in abdominal Leydig cells[18] and (2) increase in the cross-sectional area of Leydig cells in cryptorchid vs. scrotal testes.[6,17-19] In view of no significant change in total Leydig cell volume or numbers per abdominal or scrotal testis seen in the current report, some explanation is necessary to reconcile these seemingly opposite findings.

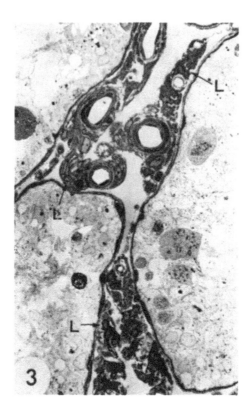

FIGURE 3.   Abdominal testis of a 2-week unilaterally
cryptorchid rat illustrating Leydig cells (L). (Magnification × 380.)

The earlier observations of Leydig cell mitoses in abdominal testes of rats made bilaterally
cryptorchid for 7 d prompted the suggestion that the Leydig cells were proliferating in
response to disruption of spermatogenesis and/or to the trophic effects of elevated serum
levels of LH. This notion was not unreasonable since at least in the normal testis, mitotic
activity among Leydig cells has not been observed[24] although interstitial cells will display
incorporation of ³H-thymidine[25] and undergo hyperplasia when stimulated chronically with
human chorionic gonadotropin (hCG).[26] In the present experiment, mitotic figures among
Leydig cells were not an uncommon feature in the abdominal testes of 7-d unilaterally
cryptorchid animals. However, it must be emphasized that within an individual animal there
was no significant change in the total numbers of Leydig cells per testis in abdominal or
scrotal testes, suggesting that if the abdominal Leydig cells were exhibiting proliferative
activity, then this phenomenon was matched by the Leydig cell population in the contralateral
scrotal testis. This data would thus favor a role for elevated LH levels as the stimulus for
Leydig cell division in the testes of unilaterally cryptorchid animals.

The discrepancy between previous observations of Leydig cell hypertrophy and those of
the present findings demonstrating no significant alteration in average Leydig cell size can
be clarified by a consideration of the methods used to obtain these data. In the past, individual
Leydig cells within the interstitial tissue were selected for measurement of their cross-
sectional area using three criteria: (1) a random selection, (2) a visible nucleus, and (3) a
clearly defined surface allowing the plasma membrane to be traced by image analysis. The
continued upgrading of morphometric technology and awareness as applied to the examination of semithin tissue sections now identifies a shortcoming in the validity of the third

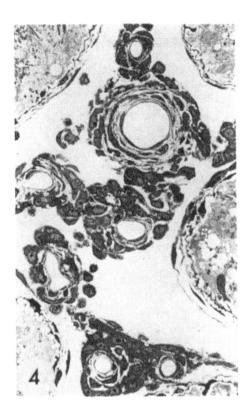

FIGURE 4. Abdominal testis of a 4-week unilaterally cryptorchid rat. Note clusters of Leydig cells surrounding blood vessels. (Magnification × 380.)

criterion. Leydig cells from a given testis are selected for the analysis of cell area only if they are sufficiently distant from neighboring cells to permit tracing their surface, while all other Leydig cells not satisfying this criterion are excluded from analysis. Indeed, as the illustrations of Leydig cell cytology clearly demonstrate, most cells do not fulfill this condition but are, to a variable extent, clustered together such that the boundaries between them are not visible by light microscopy. The alternative approach, used to obtain the present data, did not rely upon selection of individual Leydig cells. Volumetric density data were obtained by point-counting of all visible Leydig cells regardless of their degree of clustering or the presence or absence of a nucleus. In addition, estimations of Leydig cell number per testis was based upon extensive analysis of Leydig cell nuclei (and thus of cells), the amount of Leydig cell cytoplasm not contributing to the morphometric analysis.

Thus, the methods of analysis of Leydig cell morphology are of fundamental importance in the interpretation of their response to the induction of experimental cryptorchidism. Although the present observations have helped to elucidate the cytological characteristics of abdominal vs. scrotal Leydig cells, further investigation is necessary to explain the remarkable differences in their steroidogenic properties (see below) together with the contemporary concept that these changes in Leydig cell function are secondary to changes in the secretory function of the Sertoli cells.

IV. PARACRINE FACTORS AND LEYDIG CELL REGENERATION

In 1961, it was proposed that in response to experimental unilateral cryptorchidism, the interstitial cells of the abdominal testis exhibited marked hyperplasia in comparison to the

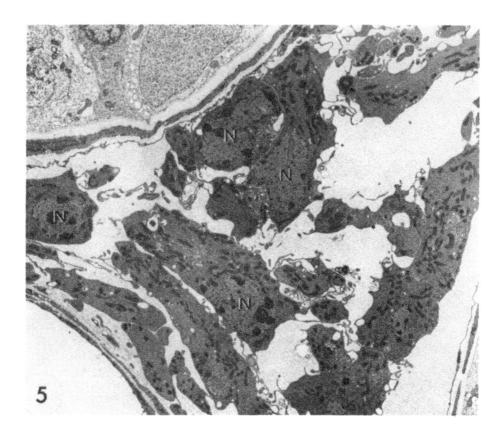

FIGURE 5. Leydig cells of the scrotal testis of a 4-week unilaterally cryptorchid rat. Note the irregular contour of the plasma membrane and the pleomorphic shape of the cytoplasm. Leydig cell nuclei (N) are shown. (Magnification × 3000.)

same tissue in the scrotal testis.[27,28] While this conclusion is now questioned by the results presented above, the same authors also reported that similar changes occurred in unilaterally cryptorchid rats which had been hypophysectomized. These observations offered circumstantial yet attractive evidence that the environment within the abdominal testis was capable of modifying the interstitial tissue in the absence of external stimulation by the gonadotropins. Recently, an alternative approach to the study of Leydig cell population dynamics has become available with the advent of the selective Leydig cell toxin, ethane dimethanesulfonate (EDS). Within 6 h of a single administration of EDS to adult rats, the Leydig cells show signs of ultrastructural alterations and between 1 and 2 d after treatment Leydig cell destruction is complete, the pyknotic debris being disposed of by macrophages.[29-31] A new generation of Leydig cells subsequently develops in the interstitial tissue, demonstrating that the loose connective tissue of the interstitial tissue is a source of Leydig cell precursors.[32,33] Judging by the pattern of Leydig cell regeneration these precursor or stem cells are located around the blood vessels and the peritubular tissues (Figures 8 and 9). With continued proliferation and hypertrophy of the new Leydig cells, they ultimately become redistributed in random locations within the interstitial tissue. The preferential association of new Leydig cells with the peritubular tissues implies that the seminiferous tubules may be a source of factors promoting the differentiation of Leydig cells. Alternatively, this observation could merely reflect dual sites of origin of new Leydig cells, namely, that perivascular and peritubular populations of mesenchymal or fibroblast-like cells proliferate and mature into recognizable Leydig cells under the influence of gonadotropic hormones. Some evidence is available to

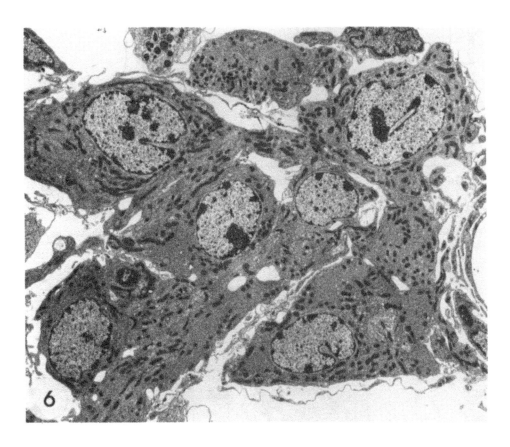

FIGURE 6. Leydig cells of the abdominal testis of a 4-week unilaterally cryptorchid rat, illustrating oval-shaped nuclei and many cytoplasmic inclusions representing mitochondria. (Magnification × 3000.)

Table 1
MORPHOMETRIC ANALYSIS OF SCROTAL AND CRYPTORCHID (CRYPT) TESTES AT VARIOUS TIMES AFTER INDUCTION OF UNILATERAL CRYPTORCHIDISM IN ADULT RATS

Morphometric parameter	Control	Duration of unilateral cryptorchidism (weeks)					
		1		2		4	
		Scrotal	Crypt	Scrotal	Crypt	Scrotal	Crypt
Testis volume (cm³)	1.2 ± 0.4	1.3 ± 0.2	0.6 ± 0.1*	1.4 ± 0.1	0.4 ± 0.0*	1.4 ± 0.1	0.3 ± 0.0*
Volumetric density of Leydig cells (%)	2.7 ± 0.7	3.0 ± 0.1	6.1 ± 0.1*	2.4 ± 0.3	7.8 ± 1.3*	2.6 ± 0.4	9.4 ± 0.4*
Total volume of Leydig cells (μl)	36 ± 5	40 ± 4	38 ± 6	34 ± 5	31 ± 6	35 ± 3	31 ± 2
No. of Leydig cells per testis × 10⁶	29 ± 1	30 ± 7	32 ± 5	29 ± 4	30 ± 2	30 ± 7	32 ± 6

Note: Mean ± SD, n = 3 animals. *, $p < 0.01$, cryptorchid vs. scrotal.

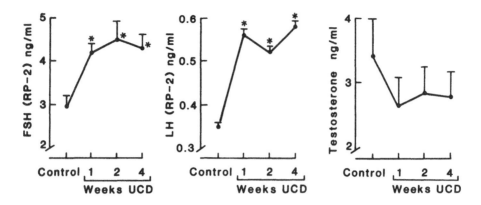

FIGURE 7.   Serum hormone levels in control and unilaterally cryptorchid (UCD) rats. Values are means ± SD. *p <0.05, UCD vs. control.

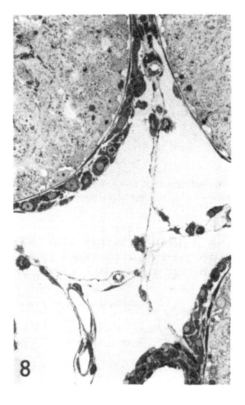

FIGURE 8.   Testicular interstitial tissue 4 weeks after EDS treatment, illustrating the peritubular distribution of regenerating Leydig cells. (Magnification × 380.)

suggest that LH alone is responsible for Leydig cell regeneration in hypophysectomized rats,[34] a finding in support of pituitary regulation of Leydig cell renewal although not excluding a role for intratesticular stimulatory factors.

The regenerative capacity of the interstitial tissue has also been examined in EDS-treated unilaterally cryptorchid rats, providing a situation in which only one testis undergoes severe spermatogenic disruption. Having eliminated the Leydig cells from the testis with EDS, the

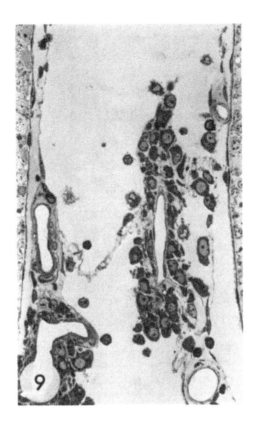

FIGURE 9. Testicular interstitial tissue 4 weeks after EDS treatment, illustrating numerous perivascular Leydig cells surrounding a capillary. (Magnification × 380.)

objective of this experiment was initially to determine if a new population of Leydig cells would regenerate within the cryptorchid testis and if so, to compare the pattern of Leydig cell regeneration in abdominal and scrotal testes. Five groups of adult rats (n = 15) received a single i.p. injection of EDS (7.5 mg/100 g body weight in dimethyl sulfoxide: water [1:3 v/v]), and a control group of 15 rats received vehicle alone. Four days later, control rats and one group of EDS-treated rats were killed. The remaining groups were made unilaterally cryptorchid and killed later at 1, 2, 4, and 8 weeks. Serum was collected from all animals and assayed for FSH, LH, and testosterone using specific radioimmunoassays described previously.[6] Testes of three rats belonging to each of the six groups were perfusion fixed with a glutaraldehyde-formaldehyde mixture, processed, and embedded in epoxy resin. Toluidine blue-stained 1-μm sections from all animals were examined by light microscopy and the interstitial tissue was analyzed using morphometric techniques.[33]

Leydig cells within the interstitial tissue of control rats showed a random distribution, at times occurring singly or in clusters. Blood vessels were often flanked by Leydig cells but Leydig cells also were seen in peritubular locations or more centrally placed within the lymphatic sinusoids (Figure 10). EDS destroyed the Leydig cells as seen in testes 4 d after treatment in which the interstitial tissue contained macrophages, endothelial tissues, and fibroblastic-type cells, but no Leydig cells (Figure 11). A similar histological picture was noted for the interstitial tissue in the abdominal and scrotal testes of the 1-week unilaterally cryptorchid rats. However, 2 weeks after the induction of unilateral cryptorchidism, the abdominal testes showed numerous fetal-type Leydig cells arranged around the peritubular tissues of the degenerating seminiferous tubules but far fewer Leydig cells were observed

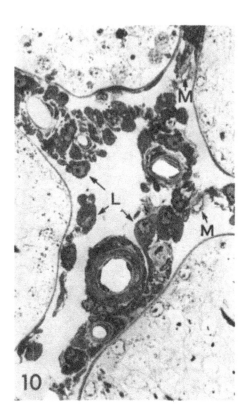

FIGURE 10.   Testicular interstitial tissue of the normal
rat testis, containing numerous basophilic Leydig cells
(L) together with macrophages (M). (Magnification ×
380.)

in the contralateral scrotal testes (Figures 12 and 13). After 4 and 8 weeks of unilateral
cryptorchidism, increased quantities of Leydig cells were seen within the scrotal testes, but
in abdominal testes the interstitial tissue contained a far greater proportion of Leydig cells
and, in particular, they were preferentially associated with the peritubular tissues of the
shrunken seminiferous tubules (Figures 14 to 17). The quantitative impression of a more
rapid regeneration of fetal-type Leydig cells within the abdominal testes as opposed to the
scrotal testes of unilaterally cryptorchid rats was confirmed by morphometric analysis (Table
2).

Despite a rapid and sustained reduction in the volume of abdominal testes, their volumetric
composition and total volume of Leydig cells per testis was significantly greater than in
scrotal testes and, moreover, proliferation of the new generation of Leydig cells was more
rapid in abdominal than in scrotal testes. Not surprisingly, serum testosterone concentrations
fell to barely detectable levels in the 4 d post-EDS group, since these animals lacked
histologically recognizable Leydig cells (Figure 18). Serum testosterone levels increased in
association with Leydig cell regeneration, but were not restored to levels found in control
animals. In response to an early decline and subsequent elevation of serum testosterone,
serum levels of LH increased significantly before returning to within the normal range at 4
and 8 weeks. A similar pattern was recorded for serum FSH, although the levels remained
elevated significantly above the control group (Figure 18). A number of conclusions can be
drawn from the observations recorded from this experiment. First, the interstitial tissue
retains its capacity to regenerate new Leydig cells regardless of whether the adjacent sem-

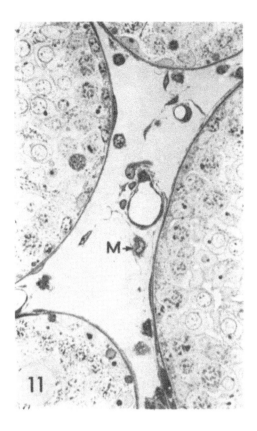

FIGURE 11. Four days after EDS treatment, illustrating interstitial loose connective tissues and macrophages (M). (Magnification × 380.)

iniferous tubules express active spermatogenesis (in scrotal testes) or severe disruption of spermatogenesis (in abdominal testes). Second, Leydig cell regeneration is more rapid in abdominal testes of unilaterally cryptorchid rats compared with that of the contralateral scrotal testes. This finding emphasizes the role of putative locally derived growth factor(s) within the cryptorchid testis which greatly stimulate Leydig cell regeneration. The exact origin or nature of these locally acting agents is not presently clear although recent evidence from the same experimental design has identified a factor in the testicular interstitial fluid which is a potent stimulator of steroidogenesis *in vitro* by Percoll-purified Leydig cells (see below and Reference 35).

The third conclusion is that there is preferential development of Leydig cells from, or closely associated with, the peritubular boundary tissues of the seminiferous tubules. In abdominal testes with very severe spermatogenic disruption, the peritubular origin of many of the regenerating Leydig cells indicates that Leydig cell precursors are located within the peritubular tissue which is thus a repository of primitive mesenchymal or fibroblastic cells capable of differentiating into Leydig cells. Therefore, it appears possible that due to their very close anatomical relationship with the seminiferous epithelium, the Sertoli cells could constitute the source of local growth factors acting on the adjacent peritubular tissue. The peritubular origin of new Leydig cells has been demonstrated in numerous laboratory species[36] and in the immature[37,38] and adult human testis.[39] A paracrine relationship between the seminiferous tubules and the interstitial tissue has been suggested by developmental studies in the immature rat testis[22,23] and by several recent biochemical studies demonstrating that these two compartments interact via the secretion of specific proteins.[1] One interesting

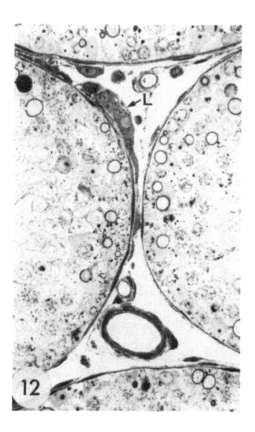

FIGURE 12.   Scrotal testis of the 2-week UCD group
after prior exposure to EDS, showing regenerated Leydig cells (L). (Magnification × 380.)

example of the specificity of this intercellular communication is highlighted by examining,
in EDS-treated rats, the relationship between the degree of spermatogenic activity in individual seminiferous tubules and the extent and pattern of Leydig cell growth which surrounds
them. As indicated in Figures 19 and 20, precocious regeneration of Leydig cells is associated
with tubules exhibiting a disrupted seminiferous epithelium, whereas few Leydig cells are
seen in proximity to seminiferous tubules with greater degrees of spermatogenic activity.
This again provides compelling evidence that paracrine interactions within the testis may be
of considerable physiological significance.

V. CHANGES IN LEYDIG CELL TESTOSTERONE PRODUCTION IN RELATION TO PARACRINE FACTORS

To assess whether the induction of unilateral cryptorchidism in adult rats resulted in
changes in Leydig cell function, Leydig cells were isolated from the scrotal and abdominal
testes of adult rats which had been rendered unilaterally cryptorchid 42 d earlier.[12] When
incubated over 5 to 20 h *in vitro*, Leydig cells from cryptorchid testes exhibited a significantly
greater steroidogenic response to hCG stimulation than did cells from the contralateral scrotal
testes (Figure 21). This change was equally evident with crude preparations of Leydig cells
(containing about 20% Leydig cells; Figure 21) and Percoll-purified cell preparations (containing about 80% Leydig cells; see Figure 23). Testosterone production by Leydig cells
from the scrotal testes of unilaterally cryptorchid rats was comparable to that for cells isolated
from the scrotal testes of normal intact rats (Figure 21).

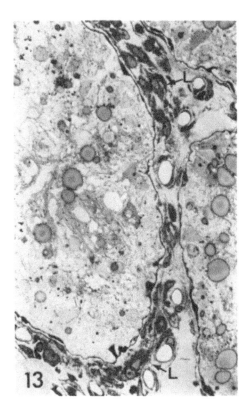

FIGURE 13. Abdominal testis of the 2-week UCD group after prior exposure to EDS, showing numerous peritubular Leydig cells (L). (Magnification × 380.)

The increase in capacity of Leydig cells from unilaterally cryptorchid testes to secrete testosterone *in vitro* is consistent with ultrastructural findings, which have shown these cells to contain increased amounts of the cytoplasmic organelles involved in steroidogenesis (see Figures 5 and 6 and above, and Reference 18). Paradoxically, this increase in steroidogenic capacity is associated with a reduction of 75% or more in the levels of testosterone in testicular interstitial fluid and spermatic vein blood from the cryptorchid testis, when compared to levels for the contralateral scrotal testis (Tables 3 and 4). Indeed, it has been suggested[7] that it is this decrease which may act as the trigger for activation of paracrine mechanisms to induce increased steroidogenic capacity of the Leydig cells in an attempt to compensate for the subnormal testosterone levels. This raises the question as to what mechanisms are activated and the cellular source of the active factor(s)?

Rat testicular interstitial fluid (IF) has been shown to contain a nongonadotropic polypeptide factor(s) which is capable of enhancing considerably LH- or hCG-stimulated testosterone production by purified Leydig cells *in vitro*,[13,40] and the levels of this factor(s) were therefore determined in the scrotal and abdominal testes of unilaterally cryptorchid rats by an *in vitro* bioassay which measures the degree of enhancement of testosterone production by purified adult rat Leydig cells incubated for 20 h with a supramaximally stimulating concentration of hCG.[13,40] The levels of the active paracrine factor(s) were increased in IF from cryptorchid testes when compared with levels in the contralateral scrotal testes or with levels in testes from intact control rats (Table 4). As judged by the dose-response effects of IF using standard parallel line bioassay methods (Figure 22) there was more than a doubling in levels of the active factor(s) in IF from abdominal testes. Similar increases in IF bioactivity

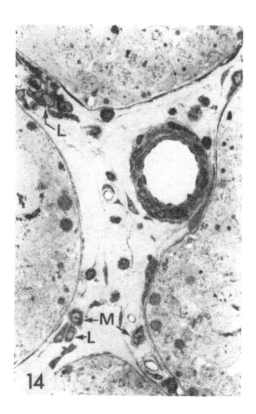

FIGURE 14.   Scrotal testis of the 4-week UCD group
after prior exposure to EDS, illustrating Leydig cells
(L) and macrophages (M). (Magnification × 380.)

have been observed in other situations in which intratesticular levels of testosterone are
subnormal[41] and/or in which there is impairment of spermatogenesis.[35,40-42] As yet the cellular
source of this IF factor(s) has not been identified unequivocally, although all of the available
evidence points to the Sertoli cell as the source of this factor.[40-42]

As yet it is not known whether exposure of Leydig cells in the cryptorchid testis to
increased levels of the IF factor(s) is responsible for inducing the increased capacity of these
cells to secrete testosterone *in vitro* in response to hCG (Figure 21), although much of the
available data would favor such an interpretation.[35,40,41] It is also noteworthy that in comparing
the *in vitro* response of purified Leydig cells from the scrotal and abdominal testes of
unilaterally cryptorchid rats, cells from cryptorchid testes not only show an enhanced steroidogenic response to hCG, but this response is enhanced to a greater degree by IF from
scrotal *or* abdominal testes, when compared to values for Leydig cells from scrotal testes
(Figure 23). Thus, Leydig cells from cryptorchid testes show increased responsiveness to
both endocrine (LH/hCG) and paracrine (IF-factor) stimuli. However, these changes appear
unable to restore normal intratesticular levels of testosterone (Table 3 and Reference 13),
presumably because the degree of LH stimulation of the cryptorchid testis *in vivo* is severely
reduced as a consequence of decreased testicular blood flow[43] and perhaps also by reduced
LH-receptor numbers.[12,44]

VI. CONCLUDING REMARKS

From the studies described above and those in the literature, it is clear that Sertoli-Leydig
cell interactions are altered in the unilaterally cryptorchid testis, although the changes may

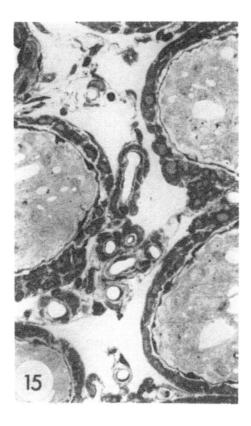

FIGURE 15. Abdominal testis of the 4-week UCD
group after prior exposure to EDS, illustrating many
peritubular Leydig cells. (Magnification × 380.)

be more subtle than those proposed to have occurred in the past, particularly in respect to
the number and morphology of the Leydig cells. The type of changes which occur in the
unilaterally cryptorchid testis are by no means unique and, in general, comparable changes
in the morphology of Leydig cells, in their responsiveness *in vitro* to LH (hCG) and in the
levels of the paracrine factor in IF which enhances the steroidogenic responsiveness of
Leydig cells to hCG, occur in other situations in which impairment of spermatogenesis has
been induced.[1] As such changes are restricted to the testis in which the impairment is present
(i.e., the contralateral normal testis is unaffected), it is generally concluded that the Leydig
cell changes are secondary to changes in the secretion, probably by the Sertoli cell, of
paracrine factors such as that present in testicular IF. These changes may in turn be secondary
to changes in Sertoli-germ cell interactions as a consequence of the removal or reduction in
germ cell numbers and/or types,[1,2] and reinforce the view that perturbation of any testicular
cell type may have 'knock-on' effects on other cell types in the testis.[1] Finally, while it is
logical, and probably correct, to conclude that the changes seen in Sertoli-Leydig cell
interactions in the cryptorchid testis reflect local changes in paracrine mechanisms, it should
be kept firmly in mind that exposure of the testis to LH and/or FSH, even in subnormal
amounts, may be necessary for these changes to become manifest.

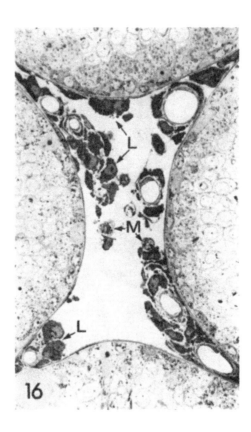

FIGURE 16.   Scrotal testis of the 8-week UCD group after prior exposure to EDS, illustrating Leydig cells (L) and macrophages (M). (Magnification × 380.)

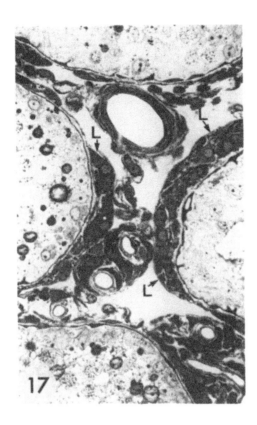

FIGURE 17. Abdominal testis of the 8-week UCD
group after prior exposure to EDS. Note peritubular
Leydig cells (L). (Magnification × 380.)

Table 2
MORPHOMETRIC ANALYSIS OF SCROTAL AND CRYPTORCHID (CRYPT) TESTES FROM RATS TREATED WITH EDS AND THEN MADE UNILATERALLY CRYPTORCHID

| Morphometric parameter | Vehicle control | Four days post-EDS | Duration of unilateral cryptorchidism (weeks) | | | | | | | |
| | | | 1 | | 2 | | 4 | | 8 | |
			Scrotal	Crypt	Scrotal	Crypt	Scrotal	Crypt	Scrotal	Crypt
Testis volume (cm^3)	1.2 ± 0.1	1.1 ± 0.1	0.8 ± 0.1	0.3 ± 0.0*	0.7 ± 0.0	0.4 ± 0.0**	0.8 ± 0.1	0.3 ± 0.0**	1.5 ± 0.1	0.4 ± 0.1**
Volumetric density of Leydig cells (%)	3.4 ± 0.2	ND	ND	ND	0.1 ± 0.0	4.1 ± 0.3**	0.9 ± 0.2	7.8 ± 0.5**	3.5 ± 0.3	20.5 ± 2.4**
Total volume of Leydig cells (µl)	42 ± 2	ND	ND	ND	1 ± 0	16 ± 1**	7 ± 2	21 ± 2**	49 ± 4	69 ± 8*

Note: ND = nondetectable, *, $p < 0.01$, **, $p < 0.001$, cryptorchid vs. scrotal. Means ± SD; n = 3 animals.

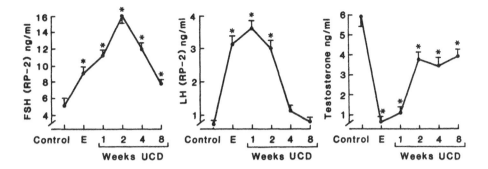

FIGURE 18. Serum hormone levels in intact control rats, rats 4 d after EDS treatment (E) and rats additionally made unilaterally cryptorchid (UCD). *p <0.05, treated vs. control.

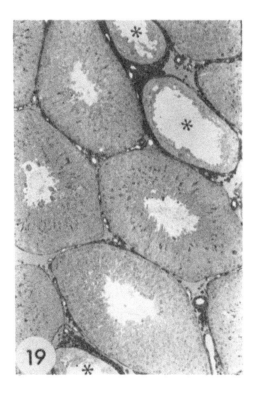

FIGURE 19. Scrotal testis of the 8-week UCD group after prior exposure to EDS. Shrunken seminiferous tubules (asterisks) exhibiting severe depletion of the seminiferous epithelium are associated with increased concentrations of interstitial cells. (Magnification × 90.)

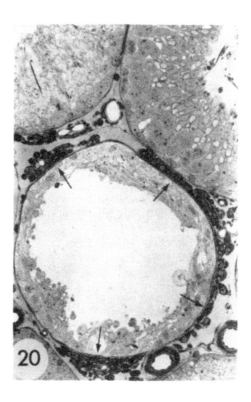

FIGURE 20.   Similar tissue to Figure 19, showing the
association between the degenerated seminiferous tubule
and numerous peritubular Leydig cells (arrows). (Magnification × 200.)

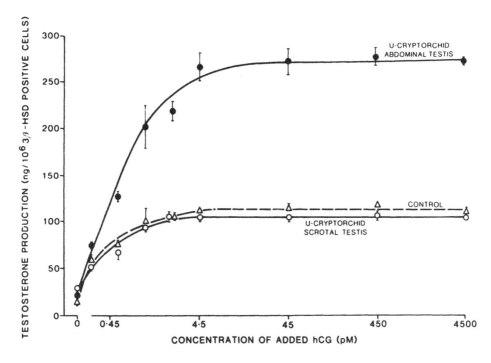

FIGURE 21. Dose-response relationship between added hCG and testosterone secretion during a 5 h incubation of isolated crude Leydig cell preparations from control rats or from the abdominal and scrotal testes of unilaterally cryptorchid rats. Each point is the mean ± SD of triplicate incubations, and results have been expressed per 10^6 Leydig cells. (From Sharpe, R. M., Cooper, I., and Doogan, D. G., *J. Endocrinol.*, 102, 319, 1984. With permission.)

Table 3
TESTOSTERONE LEVELS IN TESTICULAR INTERSTITIAL FLUID AND SPERMATIC VEIN BLOOD FROM THE SCROTAL AND ABDOMINAL TESTES OF ADULT RATS MADE UNILATERALLY CRYPTORCHID 10 WEEKS EARLIER

	Scrotal testis	Cryptorchid testis	Abdominal testis as % of scrotal testis
Testicular weight (mg)	1740 ± 136	357 ± 34*	20 ± 1%
Testosterone level (ng/ml) in Interstitial fluid	755 ± 245	67 ± 17*	9 ± 2%
Spermatic vein	87 ± 16	6 ± 1*	7 ± 1%

Note: *, $p < 0.001$, cryptorchid vs. scrotal. Means ± SD; n = 4.

Table 4

LEVELS IN TESTICULAR INTERSTITIAL FLUID (IF) FROM THE SCROTAL AND ABDOMINAL TESTES OF UNILATERALLY CRYPTORCHID RATS OF A PUTATIVE PARACRINE REGULATOR OF THE LEYDIG CELLS

Parameter	Scrotal testis	Cryptorchid testis
IF testosterone (ng/ml)	445 ± 122	357 ± 34**
Level of IF factor[a]	440 ± 95	1065 ± 228

Note: *, $p < 0.01$, **, $p < 0.001$, cryptorchid vs scrotal. Means ± SD; n = 5.

[a]   Expressed as the increment in hCG-stimulated testosterone production (ng/10^6 cells/20 h) by Percoll-purified Leydig cells induced by the addition of charcoal-stripped IF at a final concentration of 10% (for full details of the methods see References 13, 41, and 42).

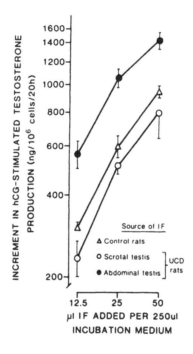

FIGURE 22.   Dose-dependent enhancement of hCG-stimulated testosterone production by Percoll-purified rat Leydig cells over 20 h *in vitro* after addition of testicular IF from either the scrotal or abdominal testes of unilaterally cryptorchid rats or from normal controls. Testosterone production in response to hCG alone was 520 ng/10^6 cells. Note that values are plotted on a logarithmic scale. (Means ± SD, n = 3).

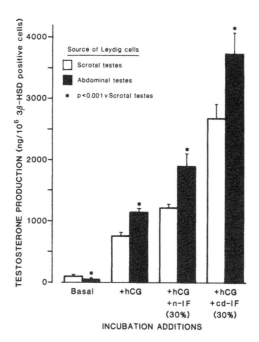

FIGURE 23. Comparison of basal and hCG-stimulated testosterone production and the response to testicular interstitial fluid (IF) of Percoll-purified Leydig cells isolated from the scrotal and abdominal testes of adult unilaterally cryptorchid rats. Note that basal testosterone secretion by cryptorchid Leydig cells is reduced whereas their response to hCG and to hCG + IF from normal testes (n-IF) or from cryptorchid testes (cd-IF) is increased compared to scrotal Leydig cells. (Means ± SD, n = 3).

REFERENCES

1. **Sharpe, R. M.,** Paracrine control of the testis, *Clin. Endocrinol. Metab.,* 15, 185, 1986.
2. **Parvinen, M.,** Regulation of the seminiferous epithelium, *Endocr. Rev.,* 3, 404, 1982.
3. **de Kretser, D. M. and Kerr, J. B.,** The effect of testicular damage on Sertoli and Leydig cell function, in *The Pituitary and the Testis,* de Kretser, D. M., Burger, H., and Hudson, B., Eds., Springer-Verlag, Berlin, 1983, 133.
4. **Nicholson, H. D., Worley, R. T. S., Charlton, H. M., and Pickering, B. T.,** LH and testosterone cause the development of seminiferous tubule contractile activity and the appearance of testicular oxytocin in hypogonadal mice, *J. Endocrinol.,* 110, 159, 1986.
5. **Fabbri, A., Tsae-Morris, C. H., Luna, S., Fraioli, F., and Dufau, M. L.,** Opiate receptors are present in the rat testis. Identification and localization in Sertoli cells, *Endocrinology,* 117, 2544, 1985.
6. **Risbridger, G. P., Kerr, J. B., and de Kretser, D. M.,** Evaluation of Leydig cell function and gonadotropin binding in unilateral and bilateral cryptorchidism: evidence for local control of Leydig cell function by the seminiferous tubule, *Biol. Reprod.,* 24, 534, 1981.
7. **Sharpe, R. M., Cooper, I., and Doogan, D. G.,** Increase in Leydig cell responsiveness in the unilaterally cryptorchid rat testis and its relationship to the intratesticular levels of testosterone, *J. Endocrinol.,* 102, 319, 1984.
8. **Bergh, A. and Damber, J. E.,** Morphometric and functional investigation on the Leydig cells in experimental unilateral cryptorchidism in the rat, *Int. J. Androl.,* 1, 549, 1978.
9. **Jansz, G. F. and Pomerantz, D. K.,** A comparison of Leydig cell function after unilateral and bilateral cryptorchidism and efferent duct ligation, *Biol. Reprod.,* 34, 316, 1986.

10. **Aoki, A. and Fawcett, D. W.,** Is there a local feedback from the seminiferous tubules affecting activity of the Leydig cell?, *Biol. Reprod.,* 19, 144, 1978.
11. **Bergh, A. and Damber, J. E.,** Local regulation of Leydig cells by the seminiferous tubules. Effect of short-term cryptorchidism, *Int. J. Androl.,* 7, 409, 1984.
12. **de Kretser, D. M., Sharpe, R. M., and Swanston, I. A.,** Alterations in steroidogenesis and human chorionic gonadotropin binding in the cryptorchid testis, *Endocrinology,* 105, 135, 1979.
13. **Sharpe, R. M., Doogan, D. G., and Cooper, I.,** Intratesticular factors and testosterone secretion: the role of luteinizing hormone in relation to changes during puberty and experimental cryptorchidism, *Endocrinology,* 199, 2089, 1986.
14. **Huhtaniemi, I., Bergh, A., Nikula, H., and Damber, J. E.,** Differences in the regulation of steroidogenesis and tropic hormone receptors between the scrotal and abdominal testes of unilaterally cryptorchid adult rats, *Endocrinology,* 115, 550, 1984.
15. **Damber, J. E., Bergh, A., and Janson, P. O.,** Testicular blood flow and testosterone concentrations in the spermatic venous blood in rats with experimental cryptorchidism, *Acta Endocrinol.,* 88, 611, 1978.
16. **Bergh, A., Asonberg, A., Damber, J. E., Hammar, M., and Selstam, G.,** Steroid biosynthesis and Leydig cell morphology in adult unilaterally cryptorchid rats, *Acta Endocrinol.,* 107, 556, 1984.
17. **Wilton, L. J. and de Kretser, D. M.,** The influence of luteinizing hormone on the Leydig cells of cryptorchid rat testes, *Acta Endocrinol.,* 107, 110, 1984.
18. **Kerr, J. B., Rich, K. A., and de Kretser, D. M.,** Alterations of the fine structure and androgen secretion of the interstitial cells in the experimentally cryptorchid rat testis, *Biol. Reprod.,* 20, 409, 1979.
19. **Jegou, B., Peake, R. A., Irby, D. C., and de Kretser, D. M.,** Effects of the induction of experimental cryptorchidism and subsequent orchidopexy on testicular function in immature rats, *Biol. Reprod.,* 30, 179, 1984.
20. **Risbridger, G. P., Kerr, J. B., Peak, R., and de Kretser, D. M.,** An assessment of Leydig cell function after bilateral or unilateral efferent duct ligation: further evidence for local control of Leydig cell function, *Endocrinology,* 109, 1234, 1981.
21. **Kerr, J. B., Mayberry, R. A., and Irby, D. C.,** Morphometric studies on lipid inclusions in Sertoli cells during the spermatogenic cycle in the rat, *Cell Tissue Res.,* 236, 699, 1984.
22. **Kerr, J. B. and Sharpe, R. M.,** Stimulatory effect of follicle-stimulating hormone on rat Leydig cells, *Cell Tissue Res.,* 239, 405, 1985.
23. **Kerr, J. B. and Sharpe, R. M.,** Follicle-stimulating hormone induction of Leydig cell maturation, *Endocrinology,* 116, 2592, 1985.
24. **Johnson, L. and Neaves, W. B.,** Age-related changes in the Leydig cell population, seminiferous tubules and sperm production in stallions, *Biol. Reprod.,* 24, 703, 1981.
25. **Niemi, M. and Kormano, M.,** Cell renewal in the interstitial tissue of postnatal prepubertal rat testis, *Endocrinology,* 74, 996, 1964.
26. **Christensen, A. K. and Peacock, K. C.,** Increase in Leydig cell number in testes of adult rats treated chronically with an excess of human chorionic gonadotropin, *Biol. Reprod.,* 22, 383, 1980.
27. **Iturizza, F. C.,** Estudios histologicas en el testiculo criptorquidico de la rata, Thesis, Universidad Nacional de la Plata, 1961.
28. **Iturizza, F. C. and Irusta, O.,** Hyperplasia of the interstitial cells of the testis in experimental cryptorchidism, *Acta Physiol. Lat. Am.,* 19, 236, 1969.
29. **Kerr, J. B., Donachie, K., and Rommerts, F. F. G.,** Selective destruction and regeneration of rat Leydig cells in vivo. A new method for the study of seminiferous tubular-interstitial tissue interaction, *Cell Tissue Res.,* 242, 145, 1985.
30. **Molenaar, R., de Rooij, D. G., Rommerts, F. F. G., Reuvers, P. J., and van der Molen, H. J.,** Specific destruction of Leydig cells in mature rats after in vivo administration of ethane dimethylsulphonate (EDS), *Biol. Reprod.,* 33, 1213, 1985.
31. **Kerr, J. B., Bartlett, J. M. S., and Donachie, K.,** Acute response of testicular interstitial tissue in rats to the cytotoxic drug ethane dimethanesulphonate, *Cell Tissue Res.,* 243, 405, 1986.
32. **Bartlett, J. M. S., Kerr, J. B., and Sharpe, R. M.,** The effect of selective destruction and regeneration of rat Leydig cells on the intratesticular distribution of testosterone and morphology of the seminiferous epithelium, *J. Androl.,* 7, 240, 1986.
33. **Kerr, J. B. and Donachie, K.,** Regeneration of Leydig cells in unilaterally cryptorchid rats: evidence for stimulation by local testicular factors, *Cell Tissue Res.,* 245, 649, 1986.
34. **Molenaar, R., de Rooij, D. G., Rommerts, F. F. G., and van der Molen, H. J.,** Repopulation of Leydig cells in mature rats after selective destruction of the existent Leydig cells with ethylene dimethanesulphonate is dependent on luteinizing hormone and not follicle-stimulating hormone, *Endocrinology,* 118, 2546, 1986.
35. **Risbridger, G. P., Kerr, J. B., and de Kretser, D. M.,** Influence of the cryptorchid testis on the regeneration of rat Leydig cells after administration of ethane dimethanesulphonate, *J. Endocrinol.,* 112, 197, 1987.

36. **Christensen, A. K.**, Leydig cells, in *Handbook of Physiology*, Section 7, Vol. 5, Hamilton, D. W. and Greep, R. O., Eds., Williams & Wilkins, Baltimore, 57, 1975.
37. **Prince, F. P.**, Ultrastructure of immature Leydig cells in the human prepubertal testis, *Anat. Rec.*, 209, 165, 1984.
38. **Chemes, H. E., Gottlieb, S. E., Pasquilini, T., Domenichini, E., Rivarola, M. A., and Bergada, C.**, Response to acute hCG stimulation and steroidogenic potential of Leydig cell fibroblastic precursors in humans, *J. Androl.*, 6, 102, 1985.
39. **Schulze, C.**, Sertoli cells and Leydig cells in man, *Adv. Anat. Embryol. Cell Biol.*, 88, 1, 1984.
40. **Sharpe, R. M. and Cooper, I.**, Intratesticular secretion of a factor(s) with major stimulatory effects on Leydig cell testosterone secretion in vitro, *Mol. Cell. Endocrinol.*, 37, 159, 1984.
41. **Sharpe, R. M., Kerr, J. B., Fraser, H. M., and Bartlett, J. M. S.**, Intratesticular factors and testosterone secretion. Effect of treatments that alter the level of testosterone within the testis, *J. Androl.*, 7, 180, 1986.
42. **Bartlett, J. M. S. and Sharpe, R. M.**, Effect of local heating of the testis on the levels in interstitial fluid of a putative paracrine regulator of the Leydig cells and its relationship to changes in Sertoli cell secretory function, *J. Reprod. Fertil.*, in press.
43. **Setchell, B. P. and Galil, K. A. A.**, Limitations imposed by testicular blood flow on the function of Leydig cells in rats *in vivo*, *Aust. J. Biol. Sci.*, 36, 285, 1983.
44. **Sharpe, R. M.**, Impaired gonadotrophin uptake *in vivo* by the cryptorchid rat testis, *J. Reprod. Fertil.*, 67, 379, 1983.

Chapter 9

CRYPTORCHID-INDUCED CHANGES IN SPERMATOGENESIS AND FERTILITY

Brooks A. Keel and Tom O. Abney

TABLE OF CONTENTS

I. INTRODUCTION

The mammal is unique in that the testis resides in a scrotum which provides a suitable thermal environment for normal spermatogenesis to occur. The testis and the scrotum together utilize a number of mechanisms to control and keep testicular temperature constant.[1] It has been known for nearly a century that increasing testicular temperature by artificial (such as applied heat, testicular insulation, and electromagnetic or ultrasound exposure) or natural means (such as cryptorchidism, varicocele, and febrile illness) results in a dramatic and often rapid diminution of spermatogenesis. The type and duration of testicular hyperthermia affect spermatogenesis and subsequent fertility differently.

The cryptorchid testis, by virtue of its ectopic location, is removed from the carefully maintained thermal environment of the scrotum and is thus exposed to relative extremes of temperature. In this section we will examine the sequelae of increased testicular temperature in terms of fertility and characterize the sites and types of cellular damage that occur as a result of thermoalteration. While emphasis will be placed on cryptorchidism, the effects of thermoalteration caused by other means will also be discussed, since the testicular abnormalities caused by these mechanisms are similar to those associated with cryptorchidism. Several excellent reviews on this subject have been presented by vanDemark and Free,[2] Lipshultz,[3] Kandeel and Swerdloff,[4] and Chapter 1 in this book. The reader is referred to these reviews for more detail.

II. EFFECTS OF HYPERTHERMIA ON SEMEN QUALITY AND FERTILITY

Perhaps one of the earliest realizations that the ectopic abdominal location of cryptorchid testes is associated with a loss of spermatogenic activity was made by Griffiths in 1883[5] in dogs. Several decades later Crew[6] postulated that a relationship existed between the higher abdominal temperature and the aspermic condition of the cryptorchid testis. About the same time, others[7-10] demonstrated that directly applying heat to the testes of guinea pigs, rats, rabbits, cats, dogs, goats, and men also decreased spermatogenesis. In many cases, a single application of heat for 10 to 30 min resulted in a marked degeneration of spermatogenic capacity.[9,11-13] Thus, even short-term increases in temperature dramatically alter the spermatogenic capacity of the mammalian testis.

The effects of artificially increasing testicular temperature in man have been studied since the early 1940s. MacLeod and Hotchkiss[14] used a fever therapy cabinet to raise body temperature to 41°C in normal males. Although no changes in sperm motility or morphology were noted, sperm production reached a nadir by 42 d and did not return to normal until 25 d later. Procope[15] also noticed that repeated use of a sauna bath produced a transient but reversible decrease in sperm numbers.

Robinson and Rock[16] observed the effects of testicular insulation on spermatogenesis by the wearing of an athletic supporter supplemented with several layers of oilcloth backed by several layers of light tissue paper. The garment was worn during the waking hours for periods of 6 to 11 weeks and ejaculates were examined weekly after treatment. A depression of sperm count occurred as early as the 3rd week of treatment reaching a nadir by the 11th week. Spermatogenesis declined to a minimum of 14% of pretreatment values by 6 weeks. Spermatogenesis recovered in about 10 to 12 weeks after termination of treatment. These investigators later observed the effects of artificially increasing testicular temperature by subjecting euspermic subjects to exposure to a 150-W electric bulb for 30-min intervals.[17] Treatment on 14 consecutive days achieved a group-mean sperm ratio (posttreatment weekly sperm count to pretreatment values) of 43.3 on the 5th week after the last treatment. Permanent recovery of sperm counts began at about the 8th week after termination of treatment. Interestingly, these results not only supported the role of increased heat as a cause of infertility but implied that this method may be applied to male fertility control.

Increased testicular temperature has also been implicated as an important factor in patients with poor semen characteristics with a varicocele, and associated with idiopathic infertility.[18] Zorgniotti and MacLeod[19] demonstrated significantly higher intrascrotal temperatures in patients with poor semen and varicocele, and certain patients with no clinical evidence of varicocele (idiopathic infertility) compared with normal men.

Artificial cooling of the testes in oligospermic men by application of an ice bag for 30 min daily resulted in increased sperm production.[17] Others have used a more sophisticated cooling device in an attempt to lower testicular temperature and increase sperm production.[20] Improvements in semen quality were observed after periods of 8 to 20 weeks resulting in increased fertility. These results suggest that the effects of increased intrascrotal temperature may be reversed by cooling the hyperthermic testis.

In a more recent study the relationships between cryptorchidism and decreased semen quality were assessed experimentally. In this study, artificial cryptorchidism was induced over a 6- to 12-month period in normospermic male volunteers by pushing the testicles up into the inguinal canal and keeping them in place each day during the waking hours by means of an adapted athletic supporter.[21] After the 1st or 2nd month of treatment, the total sperm count, concentration, motility, and motile density were significantly decreased, reaching a nadir by the 6th month. After 1 year of treatment, total sperm count declined to 12 to 34 $\times$ 10^6/ejaculate, sperm concentration declined to 3 to 10 $\times$ 10^6/ml, motility declined to 21 to 34%, and motile density declined to 1 to 3 $\times$ 10^6/ml. In men who were followed after termination of treatment, all of the semen parameters returned to the pretreatment ranges within a 6- to 8-month period. This interesting study points to the role of increased testicular heat secondary to cryptorchidism in male infertility.

The effects of increased testicular heat as a result of cryptorchidism on subsequent semen characteristics has also been examined. Fallon and Kennedy[22] found that in a group of unilaterally cryptorchid patients, sperm concentration averaged 37 $\times$ 10^6/ml; one patient was azoospermic and another was oligozoospermic (sperm count <20 $\times$ 10^6/ml). In the bilateral cryptorchid group all patients studied were found to be azoospermic or severely oligospermic (<1 $\times$ 10^6/ml). Lipshultz[3] examined sperm counts in 29 unilaterally cryptorchid patients and age-matched controls. He observed that in the postunilateral orchidopexy group, sperm counts averaged 27 $\times$ 10^6/ml compared with a mean sperm count of 74 $\times$ 10^6/ml for the controls. Eleven of these patients had sperm counts which were less than 20 $\times$ 10^6/ml. Guillon[23] reviewed a number of studies on the effects of cryptorchidism on semen quality as well as presenting his own observations. He concluded that about 50% of unilateral and only 10% of bilateral patients will have a sperm count greater than 10 $\times$ 10^6/ml. It therefore seems that spermatogenesis in bilaterally cryptorchid patients is markedly more depressed than in unilateral patients. Although paternity is increased in unilateral patients compared to the bilateral condition, semen characteristics of the unilateral patient are often found to be in the subfertile range.

A number of studies have attempted to relate the presence of unilateral and bilateral cryptorchidism with fertility. Levin and Sherman[24] and later Lipshultz[3] summarized the data to date on fertility rates in patients born uni- or bilaterally cryptorchid. Approximately 30 to 80% fertility in bilaterally cryptorchid men has been observed if orchidopexy was performed prior to puberty compared with 13% for those operated postpuberty.[24] It was suggested that if fertility was to be maintained, then the orchidopexy should be performed prior to age 10. Functionally irreversible changes in the testis appear to occur after 13 years of age.[24] However, in a more recent long-term follow-up of fertility in 64 patients treated for uni- and bilateral cryptorchidism, it was observed that 92% of unilateral and only 13% of bilateral patients fathered children, compared to 80% of age-matched controls.[22] The age at which surgery was performed did not seem to have any relationship to subsequent fertility,[22] however, the majority of the bilateral patients were operated on at 10 years or older. Gilhooley et al.,[25] in a retrospective study of 145 cryptorchid patients who had undergone orchidopexy, observed a fertility rate of 80% in the unilateral group compared with 35% in the bilateral group. These authors proposed that there may be two subsets of unilaterally cryptorchid children: a large subset which has intrinsically normal spermatogenic potential and who may exhibit germinal deficiency which is unresponsive to either surgical or hormonal treatment. This second small subset may manifest a bilateral intrinsic spermatogenic deficiency which would not be corrected by orchidopexy. According to these authors, it would be expected that the fertility of this group would not benefit from standard therapy.

Clearly, evaluation of fertility in previously cryptorchid human subjects is difficult. In an attempt to circumvent these problems, a model using experimental cryptorchidism in rats was investigated.[26,27] In these studies, Sprague-Dawley rats were treated within the first few days of life to create either mechanical cryptorchidism by suturing the testis to the abdominal wall or endocrinological cryptorchidism by estradiol administration. The ability to father offspring was assessed in these animals once maturity had been achieved. Using this model, it was observed that paternity was prevented by bilateral cryptorchidism and reduced to 45 to 60% by unilateral cryptorchidism compared to a paternity rate of 85 to 94% in sham-treated controls. Of interest was the finding that unilaterally orchiectomized rats had statistically increased paternity rates compared to the unilaterally cryptorchid group. These findings suggest that the unilateral ectopic testis may express an inhibitory influence on the contralateral scrotal testis, which may explain why many investigators have noted a reduced fertility in unilateral patients. The use of such an experimental model should shed more light on the deleterious effects of both bi- and unilateral cryptorchidism on subsequent patient fertility.

The impaired fertility associated with unilaterally cryptorchid individuals has caused some investigators to consider the possibility of an intrinsic inborn, nonreversible testicular defect associated with cryptorchidism. In an attempt to answer the question as to whether spermatogenic arrest in these cryptorchid individuals is due to an inborn testicular defect, increased abdominal temperature, or both, Frankenhuis and Wensing[28] devised an ingenious method of cooling the abdominal testis of congenital unilaterally cryptorchid boars. In this study, a twisted silicone spiral tube was attached to the tunica albuginea of the abdominal testis. Water of approximately 20°C was continually passed through the device, lowering the temperature of the retained testis 4° below that of the abdomen. After 5, 15, 25, or 45 d of cooling, the ectopic and eutopic testes were removed for histological examination. Biopsy specimens of the abdominal testis prior to the initiation of cooling revealed spermatogonia, occasional resting primary spermatocytes and, very rarely, pachytene spermatocytes. After 15 d of cooling, differentiation of spermatogonia had progressed to the formation of pachytene spermatocytes, however, no spermatids were observed. By 25 d of cooling, round spermatids were present. After 45 d of continuous cooling, differentiation of the spermatogenic epithelium had reached stage 11 in two animals, and in two other boars a few tubules containing completely differentiated spermatogenic epithelium were seen. These findings suggest that the failure of spermatogenesis to proliferate in abdominal testes, at least in boars, is due only to the increased thermal environment of the abdomen.[28]

III. SITES OF CELLULAR DAMAGE

It should be apparent from the above discussion that positioning the testis in the abdomen either by mechanical or natural means results in moderate to severe damage to the spermatogenic function of the testis. In this section we will examine studies which have addressed specific cellular damage resulting from testicular hyperthermia and we will limit our discussion to the germ cells. However, to adequately evaluate the effects of increased testicular temperature on the spermatogenic process one should also bear in mind the alterations which occur in the other cell types of the testis that directly influence germ cell development. The reader is therefore referred to other chapters in this book which deal with the effects of cryptorchidism on the Leydig cells (Chapters 3, 5, and 6), Sertoli cells (Chapter 7), and the interactions of these various cell types (Chapter 8).

As pointed out by Lipshultz[3] in his review, most of the original work on the spermatogenic potential of the undescended testis was performed by Charny and Wolgin.[29,30] These investigators presented histological evidence for three stages of normal human spermatogenic development: (1) a resting phase from birth to 4 years of age, (2) a growth phase from age 4 to 10 years, and (3) a developmental or maturational phase from age 10 years through adolescence. In the resting phase the seminiferous tubules are filled with undifferentiated cells, presumably the forerunners of spermatogonia and Sertoli cells. The tubules enlarge during the growth phase and the cells begin to take on the appearance of spermatogonia. In the maturation phase, cell division and mitotic figures are observed and spermatocytes and spermatids become noticeable.[29] It was observed that during the resting and growth phases the testis is relatively resistant to alterations resulting from cryptorchidism. At age 10, however, a lag in development of the abdominal testis can be seen. From this time onward, the longer the testis remains in its ectopic location the more pronounced the damage. Secondary degenerative changes including sclerosis and peritubular fibrosis occur, resulting in irreversible spermatogenic lesions.[30] These findings led to the conclusion that therapeutic measures aimed at correcting cryptorchidism should be implemented prior to age 10.

Mancini and others[31] reported that the cryptorchid testis showed arrest of development of the germinal epithelium and Sertoli cells which normally started at early infancy and reached a maximum in adulthood. At the time of puberty, decreased extravascular diffusion of serum proteins and fibrotic changes were noted in the stromal connective tissues and continued through adulthood. It was assumed that the arrest of development of the germinal epithelium and the progressive changes observed in stromal connective tissue are responsible for the irreparable damage observed in the adult cryptorchid testis.[31]

Similar findings were reported by Leeson[32] who performed an electron microscopic evaluation of cryptorchid and scrotal testes. In this study, no abnormalities were detected in the undescended testis prior to age 10. From this age onward, however, progressive fibrosis of the peritubular connective tissue and delayed maturation of the seminiferous epithelium were observed. Furthermore, none of the cryptorchid testes studied showed active spermatogenesis in the postpubertal period. These electron microscopic results confirmed previous light microscope findings that the undescended testis shows abnormal histologic development during puberty that becomes more pronounced in the postpubertal period.

Nearly a decade later Hadziselimovic et al.[33] provided evidence which seemed to indicate that damage to the spermatogenic potential of the cryptorchid testis may occur much earlier than previously thought. In this study electron microscopic evidence was presented which indicated that in the 1st year of life no morphological alterations of the spermatogonia were apparent in normal or cryptorchid testes. However, by the 2nd year of life a decrease in the volume density of the spermatogonia was found. Corresponding with this decrease was an increase in the volume density of degenerating cells. Based on these investigations, the authors concluded that the optimal time for surgical correction of cryptorchidism is in the 2nd year of life.[33] It would therefore appear that some histological alterations occur in cryptorchid testes as early as 2 to 5 years of age.[3]

Much of what we know concerning the effects of hyperthermia on specific spermatogenic cell types is based on the classic animal studies of Steinberger and colleagues.[12,13,34] These investigators subjected the testes of adult rats to 43°C exposure for 15 min and examined the histology of the testes at 2, 4, 6, 8, and 26 d posttreatment. It was observed that spermatogonia, resting spermatocytes, and leptotene spermatocytes up to stage XI were resistant to alteration and were able to proceed with development. Later leptotene and zygotene spermatocytes, however, showed no immediate morphologic changes but degenerated upon reaching the early pachytene stage. Pachytene spermatocytes disappeared almost completely within 2 to 6 d of exposure. Spermatids exposed in step I of spermiogenesis disappeared within 2 d while those beyond step II continued their development, although some of the resulting mature spermatozoa were retained in the germinal epithelium in stages IX through XI and were not released. These investigators pointed out that the dose of heat may effect the developing cells by interfering with one or more vital cellular functions and/or by producing a latent effect which may cause degeneration at a later stage of development. A small dose of heat may damage mainly primary spermatocytes whereas a large dose affects the development of spermatids as well.[4]

Several investigators have reviewed the effects of heat on the morphology and functionality of mature spermatozoa.[2,4,35] Kandeel and Swerdloff[4] have summarized that the evidence suggests that the extent of damage to spermatozoa is dependent upon the location of spermatozoa in the seminiferous tubule and vas deferens, susceptibility of the species to heat, and the degree of exposure. In general, younger spermatozoa which are present in the distal portions of the seminiferous tubule and in the caput epididymis are more susceptible to heat-induced alterations than the more mature spermatozoa which reside in the cauda epididymis or in the vas deferens.[4] Interestingly, the function, as well the morphology, of mature spermatozoa may be altered by exposure to heat. Functional defects include loss of fertilizing capacity, loss of motility, and a decreased survivability of embryos fertilized by heat-stressed spermatozoa.[2,4] The overall effects of heat on the spermatogenic process has been summarized by VanDemark and Free.[2] These investigators indicated that changes in temperature which adversely affect the spermatogenic function of the testis appear to affect the intermediate steps of spermatogenesis (at the level of spermatocytes and spermatids) to a greater degree than the early (spermatogonia) or final (mature spermatozoa) stages. Spermatocytes and spermatids appear to be most sensitive. Mature spermatozoa can be damaged during the stages of development in the caput portion of the epididymis. As pointed out by these authors, although the effects of increased heat may not necessarily inhibit fertilization, early embryonic development may be compromised. Therefore, although the period of heat exposure may not have been sufficient to cause noticeable changes in sperm number, those mature spermatozoa that are present in the ejaculate may be functionally impaired.

IV. THERAPEUTIC CORRECTION OF CRYPTORCHIDISM

Cryptorchidism is associated with increased risks of infertility and testicular cancer. It is deemed important therefore to take appropriate action to correct this condition in young male children. As stated earlier, some investigators recommend correction prior to 10 years of age,[24,32] while others have strongly suggested that treatment should be done by 2 years of age.[33,36] One difficulty encountered in the diagnosis of cryptorchidism is the occurrence of retractile testes. It is generally agreed that undescended testes occur in approximately 3.5% of all full-term infant males.[37] The majority of these cases are, in fact, retractile testes which spontaneously descend during the 1st year of life. Consequently, the incidence of true cryptorchidism in 1 year-olds is approximately 0.8%, essentially the same as in adult males. It has been suggested[38] that any male child suspected of being cryptorchid at birth should be reexamined at 3 months of age, and if still cryptorchid, another examination should be done at 1 year of age. Only if the testes are undescended at 1 year, should the child be considered truly cryptorchid. This rather conservative approach, if widely adopted, would probably reduce the number of unnecessary orchidopexies, estimated to be as high as 75% of the total in one study.[39]

Testicular descent is believed to involve testosterone under the control of the hypothalamic-hypophyseal axis.[37] Therefore, hormonal therapy to correct cryptorchidism has often involved treatment with human chorionic gonadotropin (hCG)[40,41] as well as gonadotropin-releasing hormone (GnRH).[42,43] In a randomized, double-blind study, Rajfer et al.[44] compared the effectiveness of hCG and GnRH in treating cryptorchid boys, ages 1 to 5 years. Several interesting observations were made in this study. First, it was observed that both hCG and GnRH therapy were relatively ineffective in promoting testicular descent in the true cryptorchid patients. Both hCG and GnRH treatment resulted in significant increases in serum testosterone levels, providing evidence of appropriate drug therapy and subsequent testicular steroidogenic response. Second, hCG treatment of a group of patients with retractile testes resulted in testicular descent in all the patients. This study suggests that short-term therapy with hCG may be a useful diagnostic technique for differentiating true cryptorchidism from retractile testes. Use of this treatment plan could also reduce the number of unnecessary orchidopexies.

If true cryptorchidism has been established through several examinations and lack of response to gonadotropin treatment, then orchidopexy is generally considered to be the correct therapeutic approach. In very young males (2 years of age or less) this procedure would be preferred over orchiectomy. Numerous studies[32,33,36] have suggested that orchidopexy at an early age may prevent some or most of the thermal-induced damage to the germinal epithelium. In this regard, several investigators[45,46] have reported similar results using an experimental animal model. These investigators demonstrated that in the surgically induced cryptorchid immature rat, spermatogenesis can be restored following orchidopexy. In contrast, spermatogenesis in the mature rat does not recover after orchidopexy.[47] Thus, age plays an important role in the subsequent recovery of the testes and development of spermatogenic capacity.

The other major concern in treating the cryptorchid patient is the increased risk of testicular cancer, particularly in the postpubertal cryptorchid male. It is generally agreed that there is an association between testicular malignancy and cryptorchidism. There is, nevertheless, controversy as to the relative risk involved and whether orchidopexy can provide a protective effect from subsequent cancer. There is, in fact, the hypothesis that a large percentage of cryptorchid testes are in fact cryptorchid because they are inherently abnormal.[48] Therefore, the association of cryptorchidism with testicular cancer may actually reflect a congenital defect in the testis which predisposes to malignancy. The relationship between cryptorchidism and testicular cancer are discussed in detail in an excellent review by Farrer and Rajfer,[49] to which the reader is referred.

Perhaps a better understanding of the physiological mechanisms which control normal testicular descent will provide insight into the causes of cryptorchidism and the appropriate strategies for treatment. Several interesting but, as yet, unproven hypotheses have been proposed in an effort to explain how cryptorchidism might occur. It has been suggested that a lesion occurs at some point in the hypothalamic-pituitary-testicular axis which interferes with or prevents normal testicular development. For example, it was shown that the levels of circulating antibodies against pituitary gonadotropin-secreting cells were significantly higher in a group of cryptorchid boys in comparison to normal controls.[50] Thus, an insufficient level of LH at a critical time in development could be an important factor in some cases of cryptorchidism. Another interesting hypothesis discussed by Hutson[51] involves a biphasic mechanism for testicular descent. The first phase, referred to as the 'transabdominal' migration, is believed to require Müllerian inhibitory factor (MIF). MIF is, of course, produced by the fetal Sertoli cells, beginning during the 7th to 9th week of pregnancy. This hypothesis suggests that testicular descent is initiated by MIF and is subsequently dependent on androgens for the second phase, referred to as the 'transinguinal' migration. Hutson et al.[52] presented an interesting model in which it was hypothesized that the effects of testosterone on testicular descent are mediated via the spinal cord and the genitofemoral nerve (GFN). The GFN then triggers development of the gubernaculum which is essential for testicular descent. Further research in these areas is certainly warranted and should provide some interesting insights into this complex area of male reproductive biology.

V. SUMMARY

In this book, we have attempted to present a rather comprehensive review of cryptorchidism and some of the basic biological alterations which occur in male reproductive function as a result of cryptorchidism. The various chapters have dealt with cryptorchidism in humans, as well as data obtained in experimental animal models. Some of the important differences in experimental models, such as bilateral vs. unilateral, and congenital vs. surgically induced cryptorchidism, as well as age differences, have been reviewed. Alterations in Sertoli and Leydig cell functions and in the morphology of these cells have been discussed. A description of the influence of cryptorchidism on pituitary secretion of gonadotropins has yielded insight into the role of the hypothalamic-pituitary-testicular axis in cryptorchidism. Throughout the book, the effects of cryptorchidism on spermatogenesis and fertility have been stressed. It is our hope that the reader has been enlightened.

REFERENCES

1. **Waites, G. M. H.,** Temperature regulation and the testis, in *The Testis,* Vol. 1, Johnson, A. D., Gomes, W. R., and VanDemark, N. L., Eds., Academic Press, New York, 1970, 241.
2. **vanDemark, N. L. and Free, M. J.,** Temperature effects, in *The Testis,* Vol. 3, Johnson, A. D., Gomes, W. R., and VanDemark, N. L., Eds., Academic Press, New York, 1970, 233.
3. **Lipshultz, L. I.,** Cryptorchidism in the subfertile male, *Fertil. Steril.,* 27, 609, 1976.
4. **Kandeel, F. R. and Swerdloff, R. S.,** Role of temperature in regulation of spermatogenesis and the use of heating as a method for contraception, *Fertil. Steril.,* 49, 1, 1988.
5. **Griffiths, J.,** Structural changes in the testicle of the dog when it is placed within the abdominal cavity, *J. Anat. Physiol.,* 26, 482, 1893.
6. **Crew, F. A. E.,** A suggestion as to the course of the aspermic condition of the imperfectly descended testis, *J. Anat. Physiol.,* 56, 98, 1922.
7. **Moore, C. R.,** Cryptorchidism experimentally produced, *Proc. Soc. Zool. Anat. Rec.,* 24, 383, 1922.
8. **Moore, C. R.,** Properties of the gonads as controllers of somatic and physical characteristics. VI. Testicular reactions in experimental cryptorchidism, *Am. J. Anat.,* 34, 269, 1924.
9. **Moore, C. R.,** Heat application and testicular degeneration: the function of the scrotum, *Am. J. Anat.,* 34, 337, 1924.
10. **Fukui, N.,** Action of body temperature on the testide, *Jpn. Med. World,* 3, 160, 1923.
11. **Young, W. C.,** The influence of high temperature on the guinea pig testes. Histological changes and effects on reproduction, *J. Exp. Zool.,* 49, 459, 1927.
12. **Steinberger, E. and Dixon, W. J.,** Some observations of the effect of heat on the testicular germinal epithelium, *Fertil. Steril.,* 10, 578, 1959.
13. **Chowdhury, A. K. and Steinberger, E.,** A quantitative study of the effect of heat on germinal epithelium of rat testes, *Am. J. Anat.,* 115, 509, 1964.
14. **MacLeod, J. and Hotchkiss, R. S.,** The effect of hyperpyrexia on spermatozoa counts in men, *Endocrinology,* 28, 780, 1941.
15. **Procope, B. J.,** Effect of repeated increase of body temperature on human sperm cells, *Int. J. Fertil.,* 10, 333, 1965.
16. **Robinson, D. and Rock, J.,** Intrascrotal hyperthermia induced by scrotal insulation: effect on spermatogenesis, *Obstet. Gynecol.,* 29, 217, 1967.
17. **Robinson, D., Rock, J., and Menkin, M. F.,** Control of human spermatogenesis by induced changes of intrascrotal temperature, *J. Am. Med. Assoc.,* 204, 80, 1968.
18. **Zorgniotti, A. W.,** Testis temperature, infertility, and the varicocele paradox, *Urology,* 26, 7, 1980.
19. **Zorgniotti, A., Sealfon, A., and Toth, A.,** Chronic scrotal hypothermia as a treatment for poor semen quality, *Lancet,* 1, 904, 1980.
20. **Zorgniotti, A. and MacLeod, J.,** Studies in temperature, human semen quality, and varicocele, *Fertil. Steril.,* 24, 854, 1973.
21. **Mieusset, R., Grandjean, H., Mansat, A., and Pontonnier, F.,** Inhibiting effect of artificial cryptorchidism on spermatogenesis, *Fertil. Steril.,* 43, 589, 1985.
22. **Fallon, B. and Kennedy, T. J.,** Long-term follow-up of fertility in cryptorchid patients, *Urology,* 25, 502, 1985.

23. Cryptorchidism, *Proc. Serono Symp.*, Vol. 25, Bierich, J. R. and Giarola, A., Eds., Academic Press, New York, 1979, 505.
24. **Levin, A. and Sherman, J. O.**, The undescended testis, *Surg. Gynecol. Obstet.*, 136, 473, 1973.
25. **Gilhooly, P. E., Meyers, F., and Lattimer, J. K.**, Fertility prospects for children with cryptorchidism, *AJDC*, 138, 940, 1984.
26. **Juenemann, K. P., Kogan, B. A., and Abozeid, M. H.**, Fertility in cryptorchidism: an experimental model, *J. Urol.*, 136, 214, 1986.
27. **Kogan, B. A., Gupta, R., and Juenemann, K. P.**, Fertility in cryptorchidism: further development of an experimental model, *J. Urol.*, 137, 128, 1987.
28. **Frankenhuis, M. T. and Wensing, C. J. G.**, Induction of spermatogenesis in the naturally cryptorchid pig, *Fertil. Steril.*, 31, 428, 1979.
29. **Charny, C. W. and Wolgin, W.**, The management of cryptorchism, *Surg. Gynecol. Obstet.*, 102, 177, 1956.
30. **Charny, C. W.**, The spermatogenic potential of the undescended testis before and after treatment, *J. Urol.*, 83, 697, 1960.
31. **Mancini, R. E., Rosembert, E., Cullen, M., Lavieri, J. C., Vilar, O., Bergada, C., and Andrada, J. A.**, Cryptorchid and scrotal human testes. I. Cytological, cytochemical and quantitative studies, *J. Clin. Endocrinol.*, 25, 927, 1965.
32. **Leeson, C. R.**, An electron microscopic study of cryptorchid and scrotal human testes, with special reference to pubertal maturation, *Invest. Urol.*, 3, 498, 1966.
33. **Hadziselimovic, F., Herzog, B., and Seguchi, H.**, Surgical correction of cryptorchism at 2 years: electron microscopic and morphometric investigations, *J. Ped. Surg.*, 10, 19, 1975.
34. **Chowdhury, A. K. and Steinberger, E.**, Selective damage induced by heat to the testicular germinal epithelium of rats, *Anat. Rec.*, 115, 217, 1963.
35. **Glover, T. D. and Young, D. H.**, Temperature and the production of spermatozoa, *Fertil. Steril.*, 14, 441, 1963.
36. **Beltran-Brown, F. and Villegas-Alvarez, F.**, Clinical classification for undescended testes: experience in 1,010 orchidopexies, *J. Ped. Surg.*, 23, 444, 1988.
37. **Scorer, C. G. and Farrington, G. H.**, *Congenital Deformities of the Testis and Epididymis*, Appleton, Century and Crofts, New York, 1972.
38. **Ansell, P., Jackson, M. B., Pike, M. C., and Chilvars, C.**, Boys with late descending testes: the source of patients with retractile testes undergoing orchidopexy?, *Br. Med. J.*, 293, 789, 1986.
39. **Cooper, B. J. and Little, T. M.**, Orchidopexy: theory and practice, *Br. Med. J.*, 291, 706, 1985.
40. **Job, J. C., Canlorbe, P., Garagorri, J. M., and Toublane, J. E.**, Hormonal therapy of cryptorchidism with human chorionic gonadotropin (hCG), *Urol. Clin. North Am.*, 9, 405, 1982.
41. **Dunkel, L., Perheentupa, J., and Apter, D.**, Kinetics of the steroidogenic response to single versus repeated doses of human chorionic gonadotropin in boys in prepuberty and early puberty, *Pediatr. Res.*, 19, 1, 1985.
42. **Hadziselimovic, F.**, Treatment of cryptorchidism with GnRH, *Urol. Clin. N. Am.*, 9, 413, 1982.
43. **Happ, J.**, Gonadorelin therapy in cryptorchidism, *Prog. Reprod. Biol. Med.*, 10, 88, 1984.
44. **Rajfer, J., Handelsman, D. J., Swerdloff, R. S., Hurwitz, R., Kaplan, H., Vandergast, T., and Ehrlich, R. M.**, Hormonal therapy of cryptorchidism, *N. Engl. J. Med.*, 314, 466, 1986.
45. **Karpe, B., Ploen, L., Hagenas, L., and Ritzen, E. M.**, Recovery of testicular function after surgical treatment of experimental cryptorchidism in the rat, *Int. J. Androl.*, 4, 145, 1981.
46. **Jegou, B., Peake, R. A., Irby, D. C., and de Kretser, D. M.**, Effects of the induction of experimental cryptorchidism and subsequent orchidopexy on testicular function in immature rats, *Biol. Reprod.*, 30, 179, 1984.
47. **Jegou, B., Laws, A. O., and de Kretser, D. M.**, The effect of cryptorchidism and subsequent orchidopexy on testicular function in adult rats, *J. Reprod. Fertil.*, 69, 137, 1983.
48. **Sohval, A. R.**, Testicular dysgenesis in relation to neoplasm of the testicle, *J. Urol.*, 75, 285, 1956.
49. **Farrer, J. H. and Rajfer, J.**, Cryptorchidism and testicular cancer, in *Principles and Janagement of Testicular Cancer*, Javadpour, N., Ed., Thieme, New York, 1986, 133.
50. **Pouplard, A., Job, J. C., Luxembourger, I., and Chaussain, J. L.**, Antigonadotropic cell antibodies in the serum of cryptorchid children and infants and their mothers, *J. Pediatr.*, 107, 26, 1985.
51. **Hutson, J. M.**, A biphasic model for the hormonal control of testicular descent, *Lancet*, 8445, 419, 1985.
52. **Hutson, J. M., Beasley, S. W., and Bryan, A. D.**, Cryptorchidism in spina bifida and spinal cord transection: a clue to the mechanism of transinguinal descent of the testis, *J. Pediatr. Surg.*, 23, 275, 1988.

INDEX

Printed and bound by CPI Group (UK) Ltd, Croydon, CR0 4YY

23/10/2024

01778245-0018